A to Z
of
Health
&Sex

A to Z
of
Health
&Sex

Dr David Delvin

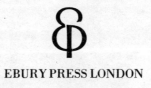

EBURY PRESS LONDON

PUBLISHED BY EBURY PRESS
an imprint of the Random Century Group
20 Vauxhall Bridge Road
London SW1V 2SA

First impression 1990

Copyright © 1990 Dr David Delvin

The right of Dr Delvin to be identified as the author
of this work has been asserted by him in accordance
with the Copyright, Designs and Patents Act 1988.

All rights reserved. No part of this publication may be
reproduced, stored in a retrieval system, or transmitted, in
any form or by any means, electronic, mechanical
photocopying, recording or otherwise, without the prior
permission of the copyright owner.

British Library Cataloguing in Publication Data.
Delvin, David
    A–Z of Health and Sex.
    1. Sex relations
    I. Title
    306.7

    ISBN 0–85223–793–6

Designed by Adrian Morris Publishing Ltd
Cover photograph Ken Browar
Transworld Features

Typeset in Futura/Bodoni by   Tek Art Ltd, Croydon
Printed and bound in Great Britain at The Bath Press, Avon

FOREWORD

"OOH DOCTOR, YOU AREN'T HALF SAUCY!"

That was the headline in the *Liverpool Echo* when they kindly reviewed my previous book in this series (A–Z of Good Sex).

And the *Liverpool Echo* was quite right. My books *are* a bit saucy, I'm afraid! But they do have a serious purpose as well – which is to help people enjoy their sex lives (and, what's more, to do it *safely*).

So here's a bit more sauce; I hope you find it entertaining.

And remember, friends: if you smoke after sex, you're probably doing it too quickly...

Dr. David Delvin

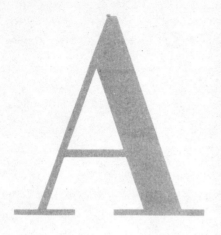

Q I'm a cabbie, and some people have the disgusting habit of holding banknotes in their mouths for a moment before they pay me. Is it possible for me to get AIDS from this?

A Well, I do agree that putting money in the mouth is a pretty mucky habit! (Talk about 'filthy lucre!').

But it would be very difficult to catch anything by accepting such a damp banknote – unless you promptly stuck it in your own mouth. Even then, I must stress that it still has not been proved that AIDS can be transmitted by saliva.

Q I have been warned against 'rimming' with my fiancé, because of the risk of AIDS.

But what actually *is* 'rimming'?

A Well, I'm afraid that 'rimming' is the exceedingly common practice of kissing and licking each other's bottoms.

Quite honestly, this practice *can't* be recommended hygiene-wise due to the fact that your *derrière* isn't exactly the cleanest part of your anatomy.

'Rimming' could give the two of

you tummy upsets, or worse, worms.

Of course, you could catch AIDS from it if your fiancé were himself carrying the HIV virus, but rather more likely is that one of you might be a carrier of hepatitis, and might pass it on in this way. So all in all, I reckon this is a bum practice. Sorry.

Q Is there any danger of catching AIDS from the water in swimming pools?

Some people pass urine while they're swimming, so presumably this might infect the water.

A Some folk do indeed have the unfortunate habit of having a pee in swimming pools.

A swimming bath technician told me that chemical tests indicate that a substantial proportion of bathers do have this rather anti-social tendency. But don't worry; the chlorine in the water gets rid of most germs – including AIDS, I hope. Nonetheless, on aesthetic grounds I would try to avoid swallowing the water from any swimming pool, anywhere!

Q I was very worried by your comments in SHE about anal sex passing on AIDS. My husband

and I do this sometimes. We have never had sex with anyone else. Are we in danger of AIDS?

A No. I've had several letters about this from worried readers. Although rectal sex is the most 'efficient' way of transmitting the AIDS virus, obviously this *can't* happen unless one of you already has it.

Q I have recently been on holiday to Central Africa and had an affair there.

I am awfully worried that this might have given me AIDS. How can I find out, without arousing my husband's suspicion?

A Well, I can't deny that you have some reason for concern, ma'am.

On the latest figures which I have available, only about 400 British women have developed AIDS after acquiring the HIV virus through intercourse.

But the majority of those caught the virus abroad – with Africa the most dangerous place of all.

So Central Africa is no place to have an affair these days! However, the odds against infection are still in your favour, and not all doctors would feel that you need subject yourself to the worry of having an HIV blood test.

Best move would be to go to the nearest large Genito-Urinary ('Special') Clinic for confidential counselling.

You live in London, and such clinics are located in all the London teaching hospitals. (You don't need a GP's letter.) Good luck.

Q I slept with a man at a party last week. What are the chances that he might have given me the HIV virus?

A At least 500 to one against at the moment – unless he was a bisexual, a drug addict, or from Central Africa or New York.

But please bear in mind that casual mating at parties is very much more likely to bring you certain other kinds of pelvic infection, such as chlamydia or gonorrhoea.

Furthermore, as we move into those 'nervous 90s' the risks of getting HIV from casual sexual dalliance will become much, much more frightening.

Q I'm a married man, but gay. I am terribly worried that I might give my wife an infection like AIDS, and I would like a check-up to set my mind at ease.

But I can't face the idea of going to one of those VD clinics and explaining to them that I am homosexual, or (I suppose) really bisexual.

A Well sir, let me reassure you that you certainly shouldn't encounter any prejudice at a clinic. What you probably don't realise is that quite a lot of clinic staff are likely to be gay themselves!

And I'm sure that, if you think about it, you'll see that there are perfectly understandable and praiseworthy reasons why they should have taken up this kind of work.

In view of your very worried state of mind, you shouldn't hesitate to go to the nearest Genito-Urinary ('Special') Clinic. They certainly won't bat an eyelid when you tell them you're AC/DC.

Q I've found out – to my great sadness – that my husband has been with a prostitute. Could this give me AIDS?

A The odds are still against it, but the risk of *other* forms of venereal infection (eg gonorrhoea) is fairly high. So it'd be best if both you and your husband went to a

Genito-Urinary ('Special') Clinic for a confidential check-up.

The fact remains that prostitutes, many of whom are drug addicts, will almost certainly soon become an important source of AIDS virus, through sharing infected needles.

Indeed, it is believed that at least one British male may have already developed AIDS through going with prostitutes, although he might have acquired the virus through sharing a razor with friends who are heroin users.

Q My mother is at home dying of cancer, and I am having to sell my body to raise the money to look after her. So I need your advice: where I can go for health checks, especially for AIDS?

A If your letter is genuine, the situation you describe is absolutely terrible. You can get special help for your mother if you ring up the Medical Social Worker at the hospital where she has been treated, and ask her to make an application to the National Society for Cancer Relief.

I'm afraid you're quite right in thinking that prostitution greatly increases your risk of catching infections – including AIDS. You can get health checks – and that includes AIDS testing if necessary

– from any of the 'Special Clinics' or 'Genito-Urinary Clinics' scattered across the country. Just ring the nearest large hospital and ask for the place and time of the next 'G-U Clinic.' Good luck.

Q My husband and I have a very good friend who is gay. I have quite often kissed him good-bye after a dinner party. Is there any danger I might have contracted AIDS?

A None whatever! With no disrespect to you, ma'am, I really am fed up with all this national panic about AIDS – and especially the way that certain people in the media have used it to vent their prejudices against gays.

I see that people have started doing crazy things like excluding gay blokes from pubs and clubs. That's bonkers! For a start, the odds against the average non-promiscuous gay having the disease are at least a thousand to one, by my calculations.

Furthermore, you *cannot* get the infection by being in the same pub, club, office, railway carriage or whatever with an infected person. All the evidence points to the fact that *very* intimate physical contact (usually actual intercourse) seems to be necessary in nearly all cases.

I've had a number of letters from gay people who are worried about the disease. And I can assure you, I didn't disappear in a puff of blue smoke when I handled their notepaper!

I'd advise any gay person who's anxious about AIDS to ring the organisation called Gay Switchboard at 01-837 7324. They are receiving around 500 calls a week about AIDS at present, and they have sensible, up-to-the-minute advice about how to avoid this disease.

Q In the mid-1980s, I had an affair with a very nice guy. It ended amicably when I got engaged to someone else. But I got an awful fright last week when I heard by chance that this former lover has been known to have homosexual leanings. Is there any chance that he could have given me AIDS?

A I'm afraid that this is a situation in which more and more women are going to find themselves over the next few years. The number of bisexual blokes around is quite incredible! So before sleeping with a man, the woman of the Nervous Nineties would do well to ask herself: 'Has my feller ever been interested in *other* fellers?'

However, in your case I don't think you've got much to worry about. I say that for two reasons:

First, at the time years ago when you slept with this bisexual chap, there had only been about 100 cases of AIDS in the country.

Second, transmission of the virus is much less likely by the vaginal route than by the rectal one.

So provided you stuck to the orthodox way of making love, it's pretty unlikely that you've acquired AIDS from this guy.

Q I have slept around quite a bit in my life. And, quite frankly, I've enjoyed it! I've slept with one or two men who probably were a bit bisexual.

Do you think the AIDS outbreak should make me put a stop to my present lifestyle?

A I fear so – agreeable though you may have found it.

Certainly, no woman in this country should ever again have an affair with a man whom she suspects is 'AC/DC'.

Sleeping with 'straight' (heterosexual) males will probably remain *relatively* free of risk of AIDS till well into the 1990s – the decade which I've christened 'the Nervous Nineties'.

By that time, AIDS will almost

certainly have hit the UK like a mediaeval plague.

Unless some miracle (like a vaccine) saves us, we're going to see death and social disruption on a scale which I find horrific to contemplate.

Q I was unfaithful to my husband three years ago, and now I have symptoms which I fear might be due to AIDS. Is this possible?

A Very unlikely, ma'am, I'm glad to say. I keep getting letters from women who are afraid that they've picked up AIDS. But I'd like to point out to all of you that at the time of writing, the total number of women in the entire country who have developed AIDS is only 150.

Sadly, this total will increase dramatically as we progress through this decade (which, sexually speaking, will be 'the Nervous Nineties', I'm afraid).

However, at the moment the chance of a brief affair giving a woman AIDS is just about nil. But if you have symptoms which worry you, then you can go to the nearest Genito-Urinary Clinic ('Special Clinic') and have free and confidential advice.

Q Is it possible for a woman to catch AIDS from having sexual intercourse with a man?

A Yes, it's possible. But it's now clear that rectal intercourse is a far more 'efficient' way of transmitting the virus. That's why about 80% of British cases so far have been male gays.

Ordinary sexual intercourse with a bloke *could* give you the germ – if he was infected with it – but you might be OK.

In practice, heterosexual intercourse with chaps will remain a very low-risk pastime for several years in the UK. But I feel that by the middle of the 1990s, there'll be so many AIDS cases around that a woman will have to think very, very carefully before agreeing to go to bed with her date.

Q I'm a gay male, and am terrified of AIDS. Where can I get some reliable information about it?

A Excellent – and frank – information leaflets are produced by the praiseworthy self-help organisation, the Terrence Higgins Trust. Send a large s.a.e. to them at *BM AIDS, London, WC1N 3XX.*

Q If a husband has been unfaithful, do you think the wife should these days demand an HIV test before taking him back?

A Well, at the moment the chances of catching HIV from a heterosexual affair in this country are still low. That will start changing now that we've entered what I christened 'the nervous 90s'.

But the current situation is that unless your husband's adultery was with a 'high risk' woman, such as a drug addict, or somebody from one of the danger areas of the world (New York, Central and East Africa – and Edinburgh and Milan), it's many hundreds to one against him having HIV. So I don't think that a test should be the most important consideration in deciding whether to take him back.

Q I was appalled by your condemnation of rectal sex. My husband and I have always found this bedtime activity very intimate and soothing, particularly when I have a period and don't want vaginal intercourse.

As we do not have AIDS, surely there is no harm in it?

A Well ma'am, I seem to have upset quite a lot of readers who occasionally go in for this practice. (In fact, 40% of women who replied to the recent SHE sex survey said they had tried it.)

Rectal intercourse between a man and woman is illegal in England and Wales – though *not* illegal for two men over 21!

There's only a risk of AIDS if one partner has the virus but there are other hygiene risks from rectal sex. Hepatitis and viral warts can be passed on, so too can an odd infection known as 'the Gay Bowel Syndrome', I kid you not!

The common practice of oral-anal contact (rimming) can transmit a form of food poisoning called giordiasis – and just possibly amoebic dysentery too.

Naturally, if neither of you are carrying these infections, then you can't transmit them.

But a word of warning: it's often common for a woman to develop a vaginal discharge if she has rectal intercourse *followed* by vaginal intercourse.

Anything that has touched bottom must *not* then be inserted into the vagina – or at least without careful washing first.

Q I am worried about getting bitten by mosquitoes when I go on holiday. Could they carry AIDS? I believe you said in SHE this was impossible. How do you know?

A I didn't say that at all! I too am a bit worried that mosquitoes which bite people who carry the AIDS virus are said to ingest the virus as they suck the person's blood.

Theoretically, it seems possible to me that a 'mozzie' could pass the virus on to the next person she bites – just as happens with malaria and yellow fever.

However, at the moment AIDS experts seem to think that this doesn't happen. The main reason why they say this is the fact that although AIDS is rampaging in Africa, very few African children have got it, thank heavens. Yet they are of course being bitten by mozzies all the time.

So, all in all, I reckon that an unwise holiday romance would be far, far more dangerous for you than a mosquito bite.

Q I have been married to my husband for 20 years, and seven years ago we went through a 'bad patch'. During that time, I am ashamed to say that I had an affair with my sister's husband. This was his only 'unfaithfulness' too.

Fortunately, we both came to our senses, and put it all behind us. I am now in love with my husband all over again.

But I am terrified that God will punish me by giving me AIDS. I am desperately upset and am losing weight fast. Could this affair have given me the virus?

A I'd say that it's virtually impossible that you could have caught AIDS from this affair, ma'am.

Your weight loss is almost certainly due to *depression*, and I beg you to see your doc and ask for help and treatment.

Actually, your letter is just one of many which I've received from women who are frightened that they may have picked up AIDS from a heterosexual affair.

I'd like to say to all of you that *if the affair was before 1985*, then it's at least a million to one against it having given you AIDS.

However *recent* heterosexual affairs are of course likely to be a bit more risky – because the AIDS virus is now so much more common.

Nevertheless, my rough calculation (based on the best figures currently available) suggests that *less than one in 200 of the sexually active population is carrying the virus.* And most of those are gay blokes.

So though the risk to women is gradually increasing, it's still quite small – except in those towns with high drug-abuse and prostitution rates, which are becoming notorious for AIDS.

Q I am a lesbian, and I wonder if it is safe for me to give blood, in view of the current AIDS scare?

A Perfectly OK. Lesbians are *not* particularly liable to AIDS – indeed, most kinds of sexual infection are rare among female homosexuals.

It's male gays who are specially liable to AIDS, particularly if they have been promiscuous in the past. Indeed, in view of recent tragedies in Australia and here – in which a number of babies and adults died after receiving blood from homosexual men – all gay males are now discouraged from giving blood.

Aids and Haemophiliacs

Re Aids and haemophilia: I've had several very worried enquiries from women whose fellers are haemophilia sufferers.

The AIDS situation for haemophiliacs and their sex partners is now very disturbing.

Haemophilia is (as most people know) the 'bleeding' disease – caused by a deficiency of a blood component called Factor VIII.

Nowadays, this vital factor can be extracted from donated blood, and given to haemophiliacs by injection so that the blood clots properly.

But thanks to a piece of what seems to me to have been unbelievable idiocy, Britain carried on importing most of its Factor VIII from America *long after the AIDS outbreak had started there.*

As a result, it is clear that over a quarter of the haemophiliacs in Britain have been infected with HIV virus.

Many of these are children, unfortunately. Others are adult males – and some of those have already infected their wives or girlfriends with the virus.

If your man is a haemophiliac, what you need to do is to join The Haemophilia Society (*PO Box 9, 16 Trinity Street, London, SE1 1DE*), and get their leaflet *Advice on Safer Sex.*

This clear and very frank pamphlet advises that you stick to the following sex rules:

Always use a sheath;
Always use *some other contraception as well* (because pregnancy MUST be avoided till you're completely certain that neither you nor your partner has the virus);
Avoid anal sex;
Don't share a toothbrush or razor (because it may transfer blood via cuts or gum abrasions).

15

ARTIFICIAL INSEMINATION

Q The doctors have advised my husband and me that we should use AIH (artificial insemination by husband) in order to conceive. But the NHS waiting list is a year long. Could we get it done privately?

A Yes, ma'am. For instance, the charity BPAS (HQ phone number Henley-in-Arden 3225) arranges AIH. They'll also advise you about a simple DIY kit which you could use at home.

Artificial Insemination

Artificial insemination is technically very easy to carry out, and has helped many couples to have much-wanted children. There are two types: AIH and Donor Insemination. In both cases the doctor simply takes some seminal fluid and injects it into the upper part of the woman's vagina at about the time of ovulation.

AIH

This means 'artificial insemination by the husband'. It's done in a few cases of premature ejaculation, and also when the husband has some anatomical abnormality which makes effective intercourse impossible.

Donor Insemination (still often known as 'AID')

This is used when the husband is completely infertile. Naturally, both husband and wife have to be completely happy that they will be able to accept a baby which was really fathered by another man.

It's also important to realise that Donor Insemination is far more contentious than AIH. It's illegal in some countries, and in *all* countries there may be legal problems about registering the parents' names on the child's birth certificate. Relatives and friends may not be too understanding, so most AID couples keep quiet about it.

In general, what happens is that the doctors or clinic who are providing the service have a list of donors — who are frequently medical students. Obviously, the chosen donor should roughly match the husband in general colouring, race and physical size. You will have to rely on the doctor or clinic for this —

16

Q My husband is completely infertile, so it looks as though my only hope of having a baby is by artificial insemination. Do you think I could do this without telling him? And, if so, where could I get it done?

A To have artificial insemination by donor without telling your husband would be utter lunacy!

For a start, he presumably *knows* that he's completely infertile. He might just suspect something when

because it's almost unknown for the donor to be introduced to the couple. In most countries, the doctor will attempt to keep the man's identity a complete secret, though it has been suggested that proper registers of donors should be set up, so that the name of a donor could, if necessary, be checked at a later date.

Some doctors working in the field have allowed individual donors to father many children through insemination. But it's now increasingly felt that a young man who is a sperm donor should make only a few 'donations', *not* in order to save his strength for his medical studies, but to cut down on the risk of inter-marriage among the children he has sired.

There's now increasing emphasis on screening potential sperm donors to make sure that they're healthy (and don't have

AIDS). But you have to bear in mind that in the unlikely event of the baby being born with some abnormality, there's no question of your having any legal redress, unless there has been some form of negligence.

As with AIH, the procedure for carrying out AID is very simple. The selected young man arrives at the clinic, and makes his 'donation' into a sterile container. It may be immediately frozen for use later. But it's possible that the doctor will have arranged for the donor to donate on the day that you're due to ovulate. You will come to the clinic a little later in the day, and the doctor will use a syringe to inject the sperm into the upper part of your vagina (the area of the cervix).

you announce that you're in the family way. What he'll probably suspect is that you've been up to no good with the lodger!

No, if you're considering insemination then it can only be with your husband's agreement. A high proportion of infertile men *will* agree, if their wives talk it over with them carefully.

Q My husband has been told that he is completely sterile, so we have decided to have a baby by AID. Where can I get more information about this?

A You can get a leaflet about AID from BPAS – phone number 01-222 0985.

Q I have a BO problem. People in the office have complained, and I feel that if I had a sexual relationship with a man, he would too! I've tried everything my doctors have suggested. Can you help?

A As a rather drastic solution, there is an operation to remove a saucer-sized area of skin from the armpits. This works very well – but it's painful!

Less drastic is a new invention for which great claims are being made. It's a battery-operated device which you place on the appropriate part of your body. The makers claim that it produces a temporary blockage of the sweat ducts, but you have to re-treat yourself every six weeks or so.

At present, it's unlikely to be available on the NHS, and it's pricey – £98 for the armpit model. More details from: John Bell and Croyden Ltd, *52–54 Wigmore Street, London W1H 0AU.* I wouldn't myself recommend buying such a device without clear proof that it works.

Q I read what you wrote about female baldness – pubic and otherwise. (See also PUBIC)

I'm a young woman and have suffered a lot of distress because of severe hair loss on my head. Is there any self-help group for sufferers?

A Yes: write (enclosing a large s.a.e.) to Hairline International, *Hill Vellacott, Post and Mail House, Colmore Circus, Birmingham, B4 6AT.* They're a support organisation for adults and children who've lost their hair.

I do hope that the new treatment called minoxidil (Regaine) will be able to help you get some of your hair back.

Q I am desperately shy. In fact I cannot even let my own husband see me without any clothes. My doctor said something called 'behaviour therapy' might help. Please can you explain more about this?

A Well, she's right. Behaviour therapy is a specific system of treatment which concentrates on helping you to find ways of altering your symptoms – rather than digging around in your Freudian past! I've seen behaviourist seminars at which shy people are taught how to modify their own reactions – by role-plays, etc. And I'm sure the same thing could be done for your shyness about undressing. Your 'role-plays' for this could be quite something!

Q My husband's sperm has gone red. Is this OK?

A No, ma'am. This suggests that there's *bleeding* somewhere in his plumbing, and it must be investigated *soon*.

Your doctor will probably suggest that he goes to a urological surgeon for the necessary tests.

Q I have been a widow for five years, and have recently embarked on a love affair. After intercourse, I've been surprised to note a pink/red secretion. Is this just due to me being unaccustomed to lovemaking, or should I talk to my GP?

A This was almost certainly blood, and therefore you'd be best to have a check-up from a doctor. Indeed, *anyone* who bleeds post-coitally (especially after the menopause) would be wise to see her doctor.

But as you say, this may just have been due to the fact that you're a trifle out of practice. If so, a simple lubricant like KY or Durol (available at most chemists) would help until you've played yourself in.

Q I am 19 and since I lost my virginity a year ago, I have had (a) bleeding after every intercourse; (b) a yellow bubbly discharge, which has not got better on anti-thrush treatment from my doctor.

A The yellow, bubbly discharge is likely to be due to the infection called trichomonas. If your doc agrees, he/she will probably give you Flagyl tablets by mouth. Persistent bleeding after sex usually needs specialist investigation, but at your young age it is unlikely to be due to anything nasty.

Q I have recently heard of 'cystic breast disease'. As I have a hard lump in each breast, just below the nipple, I feel I may have this. Do you think so?

A I beg you to see your doctor *urgently*. There's no way anyone can diagnose breast lumps except by examining them. Most likely these lumps are benign, but you *must* make sure.

This month I have several letters in my postbag from women who say they have breast lumps. The vital message which *every* woman should know is this: if you think you've noticed a lump in the breast, *always* have it checked out within a few days at most. Doing this could save your life.

Q I have what I think must be a fairly unusual complaint — my breasts are different sizes. I have met a man who I really care for, but I feel embarrassed at the thought of undressing in front of him. I have neither the means nor the inclination to submit to plastic surgery, so what can I do?

A This isn't all that unusual a problem. Many women have one breast which is much bigger than the other. But I do appreciate that this is deeply embarrassing for you. Really, the only cure would be by plastic surgery — which you might be able to get on the NHS.

If surgery's not your cup of tea, then you might be able to produce at least a slight improvement by regular and intensive exercise to build up the muscle behind the smaller breast.

The simplest way of doing this is just to put your hand on your hip bone, and press down very hard for about ten seconds. (This makes the muscle behind your breast stand out.) Relax for a few seconds – then repeat ten times.

As with any muscle-building exercise, you need to do it night and morning for about six months before you get any results. Very good luck to you.

Q My breasts are very small. Would hormone pills help?

A No – don't muck about with hormone pills, which could be dangerous. Really, the only way in which anyone can make any really significant increase in her boob size is through cosmetic surgery.

Q My teenage daughter has been horrified to discover that at the same time as her breasts developed, a third breast has appeared on the lower part of her chest. There has always been a little brown mark on her skin there, but it now appears that this was a nipple.

We haven't told anybody else yet. Can anything be done?

A Please try and reassure your poor daughter that this condition is quite common, and can be very easily put right.

Having more than two breasts is called 'polymazia'. Famous sufferers have included Anne Boleyn, who is said to have had three. A woman whose case was recorded in a Victorian medical journal had nine, and another had an extra breast on her thigh!

But why does it happen? Look at a cat or a dog, and you'll see. They have a double row of teats, running down the chest and the abdomen. And just like them, human beings also have a streak of embryonic tissue which is called the 'milk line', which runs from the top of the chest down to the groin.

These extra nipples are perfectly harmless. But sometimes at

The Breast

The breast is a structure which, as you know, has always had enormous emotional importance for human beings. That breasts were regarded as supremely beautiful way back in Old Testament days is evidenced by the Song of Solomon: 'Thy two breasts are like two young roes that are twins, which feed among the lilies . . .'

To this day, men have tended to be obsessed with breasts; Freud (1856–1939) believed that boy babies learned their sexuality at their mothers' breasts, and that this explained the male fascination with the mammaries. (Where this leaves bottle-fed boy babies – and indeed girl babies – I don't know.)

Structure

Anyway, let's have a quick look at the basic anatomical structure of the human mammary.

The breast is a mass of milk gland tissue, embedded in fat, and set on the front of the muscular wall of the chest. From the glands which produce milk, a number of milk ducts (15 to 20) lead down to little milk sinuses (or collecting areas) just behind the nipple. In between the milk ducts, there's a network of fibrous tissue which gives the breast support – and also gives it that

puberty one of them develops into a full-blown breast – which is what has happened with your daughter. Happily, this unwanted extra breast can be surgically removed. That's a job for a plastic surgeon, and your GP will be pleased to refer your daughter to one under the NHS.

Q I am 19, and have just found a lump in my right breast. Is this cancer?

firm, thrusting outline so beloved of adult males and babies. This fibrous tissue does tend to stretch with advancing years, particularly if the breasts are very big and heavy.

Size of the breasts depends on the amount of fat and glandular tissue contained in them, which is to a large extent controlled by the woman's own hormones. It's difficult and dangerous to achieve any change in breast size by giving hormone treatment. But nowadays it is not difficult to enlarge abnormally small breasts (or to reduce abnormally large ones) by plastic surgery.

A At your age, breast cancer is fantastically rare. (See page 24.) But any lump in the breast, at any age, should be examined by a doc.

Q As I've been on the Pill for four years, am I in danger of developing breast cancer?

A Research about the Pill and breast cancer is coming in very fast at the moment. Most of it is fairly reassuring, but there are disturbing suggestions that prolonged exposure to the Pill in younger women (especially those who have never been pregnant) may – and I repeat *may* be linked with breast cancer. But there are two factors which make it very difficult to assess th figures.

Firstly, the majority of cases of breast cancer occur in women aged 55-plus. At the moment, very few women over 55 have had much exposure to the Pill.

Secondly, in the case of most carcinogens (cancer-provoking agents), there's a 'time-lapse' of about 25 years after exposure, before the cancer occurs.

This means that because the Pill was scarcely used in Britain before about 1965, we wouldn't expect to see many Pill-induced cancers appearing till about now. ▶

So I'm afraid we shall soon find out whether the Pill turns out to have been a boon to womankind – or the proverbial biological time-bomb.

AGE	CASES PER YEAR
15–19	1
20–24	15
25–29	107
30–34	376
35–39	750
40–44	1288
45–49	1744
50–54	1969
55–59	2411
60–64	2371
65–69 (PEAK)	2754
70–74	2575
75–79	2131
80–84	1472
85+	1200

Q I have just had a course of radiotherapy treatment following a 'lumpectomy' operation to remove a tumour from my breast. I am now feeling well and have been declared fit. But I am writing to make the point that when I first realised that I had a lump, I did not rush to the doctor (as I had always sworn that I would do in such circumstances). Indeed, when my doctor gave me a referral form to take to the hospital, I waited for a while before sending it off.

Disorders of the Breast

Cancer

What happens if you consult your doctor because you think you have found a lump? He will, of course, examine you himself to confirm that one is present. (Some women understandably mistake a slight thickening of the breast tissue for a lump.) Having assessed the swelling, he will arrange an urgent referral to a surgeon, who will usually perform a minor diagnostic operation on the breast within a few days.

This operation may just involve aspirating some fluid from the swelling with a needle – or it may involve taking away a tiny portion of the lump for examination under the microscope. These procedures will show if cancer is present. If it is, treatment will be started immediately.

The treatment of early breast cancer is nowadays fairly successful. This isn't the place to discuss the merits of the various methods of surgery and radiotherapy. Suffice it to say that the woman who has gone to her doctor *immediately* she has discovered a lump stands an excellent chance of living to a healthy old age.

Women tend, quite naturally, to be very frightened of the idea of losing a breast, but the courage that most women show in the face of this disease is quite remarkable.

N.B. Although breast cancer almost always makes its appearance in the form of a lump, it can sometimes cause other symptoms instead. The most common are *(i)* bleeding from the nipple, *(ii)* recent (as opposed to lifelong) inturning of the nipple, *(iii)* puckering of the skin of the breast, *(iv)* a raw, weepy area developing on the nipple.

Other Breast Conditions

SWELLINGS. There are many benign causes of lumps in the breast but, as explained above, tissue from all such lumps must be examined under the microscope within a matter of days. Removing a benign lump is a simple matter, and no further trouble need be anticipated after the operation.

OVER- AND UNDER-SIZED BREASTS. Many women are understandably dissatisfied with the size of their breasts. Where the bosom is very big or small, plastic surgery can sometimes help. Hormone creams should not be used, as they are dangerous. Many proprietary 'bust-developing' preparations are completely useless. The most popular 'bust-developer' in the world is, in fact, a simple exerciser, the object of which is to develop the muscles that lie behind the breast. It has at least the merit of being harmless!

MASTITIS. This means inflammation of the breasts. Most types of mastitis are fairly trivial, and respond moderately well to simple measures, such as wearing a better-fitting bra. Infective mastitis, however, will need antibiotic treatment and may progress to the stage of a breast abscess (*see* below).

BREAST ABSCESS. This is a common condition, at least during lactation. A painful swelling develops in the affected breast, and the overlying skin becomes reddened. Surgical opening of the abscess may be necessary, but in the early stages antibiotics alone may be sufficient.

When my lump was eventually diagnosed as malignant the trauma was made worse by my feelings of anger with myself for not having acted with more urgency. I know that 'putting it off' is the most natural human reaction in such circumstances. But I am writing to urge you to continually remind your readers of the need for regular and constant self-examination, and the importance of getting treatment *immediately*, even if the doctor says (as mine did) 'It's probably nothing!'

AQuite right ma'am. There's nothing further to add to the point you have made so eloquently – so I'll just salute your courage, and thank you for taking the trouble to put this potentially life-saving advice on paper for the benefit of other readers.

QI am 31, and very worried about cancer of the breast. I'd like to have a mammography screen, but my GP says the NHS can't afford it. Is this true?

ARegrettably, mammography (which is X-ray screening of the breast) isn't easily available in some areas of the country. But it is

Women: Care of Your Breasts, and Protecting Yourself Against Cancer

General care of the breasts isn't difficult: a straightforward wash with mild soap and water once a day is sufficient, followed by careful drying with a soft towel.

In late pregnancy and more especially early lactation, breasts and nipples need special care – mainly because cracks are liable to develop in the nipple. In the event of any cracking or soreness, apply a reliable antiseptic cream (your local pharmacist will advise you). If pain or even appreciable soreness develop, always consult your doctor or midwife.

Breast Cancer

It's a tragic and, to most people, unpalatable fact that breast cancer attacks roughly 1 out of every 17 women in western countries. (I can't help feeling that if cancer of the penis were as common in men, something would have been done about it by now!)

Many of these cases of breast

cancer can be cured if caught early enough. X-ray screening for women is gradually being introduced. But at present it is only for the 50–64 age group. The fact is that for most women the best hope of catching the disease early is to detect it themselves.

Possible warning symptoms are:

a *lump* (this may well not be cancerous, but should *always* be checked by a doctor)

much less commonly, unexplained *bleeding* from the nipple

occasionally, a *raw ulcer-like patch* of skin on the nipple

sometimes, an unexplained *inturning of the nipple*

unexplained *puckering of the skin* of the breast.

I should add that although many teenage girls and young women not unreasonably fear that they have breast cancer, it's primarily a disease of the over-

30s – and is commonest in the over-50s. Cases occurring before the age of 25 do occur, but are very rare indeed.

The process of monthly self-examination for breast lumps is vitally important. (I'm not joking when I say that husbands and lovers can help here too, by looking out for lumps when they handle their loved ones' breasts.) An examination once a month should be sufficient. Feel all over the breast tissue, using the flat of the hands. If there is any lump present, **see your doctor within 24–48 hours.**

This breast check, should be a regular self-examination. The procedure is based on the splendid and underfunded work of the Women's National Cancer Control Campaign in Britain. An excellent leaflet describing the technique is available from WNCCC at *1 South Audley Street, London W1Y 5DQ* – enclose a large s.a.e. Follow it: it could save your life.

supposed to be coming in for all women between 50 and 65.

If you feel you'd be happier having it done, then all I can suggest is that you ask your doc to refer you to one of the large private screening units run by organisations such as BUPA.

But let me make one important point. Few people have grasped that regular routine mammography only appears to be of value in women aged over about 45.

At the present moment, the best and most available defence against breast cancer for younger women seems to be to keep on examining your breasts for lumps once a month.

And of course, if you have the slightest suspicion of a lump – or anything else odd – in your breast, then I beg you to get a medical examination right away. Recent work suggests that many women are still waiting six or seven months before seeing a doctor – by which time it may be too late.

Q Although I like having my breasts handled, I am seriously concerned that this sort of manipulation could lead to breast cancer. Is this so?

A Fortunately, it's just a myth. Women who have their breasts handled a lot are *not* specially liable to breast carcinoma. For example, the incidence of this awful disease is far less in prostitutes than it is in nuns.

Q As a birthday present, my husband is going to pay for me to have plastic surgery to make my boobs bigger. Where could I get this done?

A Who's the birthday present for – you or him?

If you really want this done then good luck to you. However, it's important for you to realise that plastic surgery on the breast isn't always as successful as people think; so it's always best to go to a top-class, reputable plastic surgeon.

Where are you going to find one? Personally, I wouldn't recommend going off to one of the cosmetic surgery clinics which advertise in newspapers – unless you know that the clinic in question has a good local reputation. Nobody really controls the standards of these clinics, and some have been known to give people cross-eyed boobs!

Some clinics claim that they are 'approved by the Area Health Authorities' – which means virtually nothing. Others announce that they only employ Fellows of the Royal College of Surgeons – which again doesn't mean much, because you don't need to have done any plastic surgery at all to become an FRCS.

So what's to be done? My own view is that in most instances it's best to begin by asking your own doc to refer you to a plastic surgeon. Though you'll obviously have to go privately, your GP might well choose a surgeon who is a consultant in plastic surgery at an NHS hospital. (Being a consultant at a large hospital is obviously a considerable guarantee of ability.)

Alternatively, there are now two organisations of surgeons who do this kind of work. If your doc doesn't know the address of a plastic surgeon, he or you can write to either of these organisations to obtain a list of names and addresses.

The two organisations are:

• The British Association of Aesthetic Plastic Surgeons, *c/o* The Royal College of Surgeons, *Lincoln's Inn Fields, London WC2A 3PN.*
• The British Association of Cosmetic Surgeons, *c/o 7 Patterdale Road, Woodthorpe, Nottingham NG5 4LF.*

Q I have always had one breast that is much, much smaller than the other, which has caused me terrible embarrassment. I have now been offered the chance of plastic surgery to implant a 'pad' into the smaller breast and make them the same size. Should I go ahead?

A Yes. All surgery carries a slight risk. But if you really feel bad about the fact that you're a bit like the young lady of Devizes (whose boobs were of differing sizes), then go ahead and have the op.

Q For all my adult life I have been deeply unhappy about my almost completely flat chest. (Currently, I have difficulty filling a 30AA bra.) Small fortunes spent on creams and potions and hours of 'bust-building' exercises have been to no avail. For many years now I have thought about having a boob job done, but the high cost made this an impossibility. However, I am finally in a financial position to afford it. How can I go about finding a good cosmetic surgeon? Please don't tell me to forget all about it, or start expounding the everybody's beautiful in their own way theory!

BREAST IMPLANTS

A I wouldn't dream of it: flat boobs can make a woman feel as though nature's dealt her a lousy hand. However, I'm not too happy about some of these cosmetic surgery clinics which advertise to the public; you may end up getting your breasts operated on by a dentist (seriously), so write to the addresses on the previous page.

Q A few years ago I had breast implants to increase my bust size. It was one of the best things I've ever done, and has given me great self-confidence.

But this year I'm going on holiday abroad, and will be flying for the first time. Is it true that people who have had breast implants should not fly, because the implants can explode at altitude?

A In the early days of breast enlargement, there were one or two reports of implants going 'pop' when the airliner reached about 40,000 feet. But this just doesn't seem to happen today – perhaps because surgeons use a better class of implant.

However, I should point out to you that 'falsies' (inflatable brassières filled with air) can and do explode in the low-pressure atmosphere of an aircraft. Travellers who rely on pneumatic devices to boost their bustlines should discreetly let out a little air in the Departure Lounge.

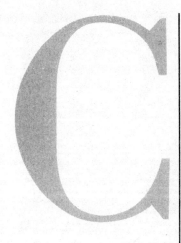

Q I am getting fed up with the Pill, which makes me feel depressed and bloated.
Is the cap any good?

A Yes, jolly good method, the cap. If you use it properly, it's nearly as effective as the Pill.

Also, it has practically no side effects — except that urinary infections (like cystitis) seem to be more common in cap-users.

All Family Planning clinics fit caps, so get yourself down there and get measured up for one of the correct size.

Q You will probably think me very haughty, but I do have several lovers, who do not know about one another. For contraception, I rely on the cap. Would it be better if I used a different one for each lover?

A Goodness, you do seem to be living life in the fast lane. Anyway, the cap (diaphragm) is designed to fit the woman — not the man. So there is no need to have a separate one for each gent.

Perhaps you were worried about the hygiene of using the same diaphragm for each man? As a rule, most women take out their caps about eight hours after intercourse, then wash and dry them.

This procedure will give perfectly adequate hygiene, provided you can fit it into your schedule.

The Cap (Diaphragm)

The cap or diaphragm has become more popular in recent years, probably as a result of various pill scares. The most widely used contraceptive cap is a simple disc of rubber. The idea is that a woman slips it into her vagina *so that it covers her* cervix (the neck of her womb). Before putting it in, she coats it with a contraceptive cream or gel.

Rather surprisingly *neither she nor her partner should be able to feel the device once it's in position.* So a well-fitted cap shouldn't interfere with love-making in any way.

The important words here are 'well-fitted'. Women's vaginas vary substantially in size, so you must be fitted (by a doctor) with the size of cap which is right for you. Equally importantly, you

have to be taught how to put the device in correctly before love-making, and how to take it out the following morning.

The cap *must* be inserted so that it covers the cervix – otherwise it will be quite useless.

When the cap fails to protect against pregnancy, the usual reason is that the woman has been putting it in the wrong place – usually in *front* of her cervix. So it's very important to be sure that you understand your own anatomy before you rely on this method.

Note: there are some rarer types of cap available in Britain and other countries (not widely in the USA) for women whose vaginal muscles are too lax for an ordinary diaphragm. Several new types of cap have also been invented recently.

Q I had six or seven lovers when I was younger, including a couple of 'one-night stands'. I presume from what I have read that this means I am likely to get cancer of the cervix. Am I right?

A No, ma'am – you're not. I keep trying to make clear in this column that cancer of the cervix *isn't* just 'caused by sex', as you might think from reading some newspapers.

It appears to be linked with a number of factors, which include the pill, smoking, social class, geographical location, race – and whether your partner (or possibly yourself) is involved in ·manual labour.

In other words, it's still a mystery! But certainly, your chances of developing it are increased if: (a) You've had multiple sex partners; or (b) Your husband has had multiple sex partners.

In your particular case, the fact that you've had what us doctors euphemistically describe these days as 'a number of boyfriends' *doesn't* mean that you're certain to get cervical cancer – though, like everyone else, you should have regular smears.

One final point: the current publicity over cancer of the cervix has led many people to think, like yourself, that the chances of dying from it are high.

This isn't so. One woman in 150 dies from cervical cancer. One woman in every 30 dies from lung cancer – and one in every 23 from breast cancer.

The last two are REALLY common causes of cancer deaths in women, and it's a great pity that more isn't being done to prevent them. (If I were prime minister, I'd start off by jailing a few tobacco manufacturers!)

Q My ex-wife has developed cancer of the cervix.

I'm very worried about the theory that this is caused by a germ. Could I have transmitted it to other women I've made love to? And should I contact them to warn them?

A That's very thoughtful of you. The 'germ theory' of cancer of the cervix is still unproven. Also, if you have been a reasonably hygienic chap (in other words, if you wash your penis each day) that lessens the chance of having passed anything on.

But I think it'd be reasonable if you indicated to your lovers – without alarming them – that they should have regular smear tests. If they do that it's very unlikely that they'll be in danger.

Q I am in my mid-30s and have just had a routine smear which revealed I have 'mild dysplasia'.

The doctor told me that this is the

pre-cancerous phase. I am feeling very unhappy, and wondering how my husband and small children will manage without me when I am gone.

How can I have got this cancer, as I thought it related to promiscuity? I have never slept with anyone apart from my husband.

A First thing to say, ma'am, is that there has been some massive misunderstanding here. You have nothing to worry about, and are not going to die.

'Mild dysplasia' is a common finding, which means that the cells could well become cancerous if left long enough. They may get better over the next few years – but if they don't, a simple operation will cure you. So cheer up!

Second thing to say is that a lot of people seem to have got this idea that you can't get cancer or pre-cancer unless you've slept around. That's a load of old-rhubarb (as we doctors say).

There are other factors, such as smoking, having had several babies, and being married to someone in a manual job.

Q I work in a hospital cytology department, and I noted with interest your comments on cervical screening in SHE (in which you complained about the lack of availability of smear tests for British women).

Surely the majority of women who die from cervical cancer have not had the test because they did not come forward for it – and not because the test was unavailable to them?

A I must admit, sir, that there's some truth in what you say: many women have the opportunity of having the smear test, but either refuse it or else don't bother.

On the other hand, there are plenty of women who have great difficulty in getting a smear done. And there are a lot of others (particularly in the poorer areas of Britain) who've never had a smear because our creaking NHS has never offered them one.

Q Would my doctor remember to let me know if my smear test showed cancer? I have always had regular smears, and thought I was safe. But I have been horrified to read that women may have died because doctors didn't tell them their test results.

A Well, I've been saying for years in SHE that our national smear test system is a muddle and

The Cervix

Every woman should be familiar with her own cervix – after all, if a man can touch your cervix, why shouldn't you?

But, what *is* the cervix?

As you probably know, it's widely referred to as 'the neck of the womb'. But really it's the *tip* of the womb, the very point of the womb, which projects down a few centimetres into the vagina.

A narrow tunnel runs up through the cervix and into the cavity of the womb itself. This is the only way into the womb from the exterior. Sperms pass up through this canal into the womb immediately after intercourse. Naturally, menstrual blood passes down through it at period times.

And, of course, during childbirth the baby has to pass through this hole through the middle of the cervix. Fortunately, the cervix has the remarkable property of opening up to a quite extraordinary extent during labour – so that the previously-narrow tunnel becomes wide enough to let the baby's head go through it. (It shrinks' down almost to the same size as before, very soon after childbirth.)

Functions

It's difficult to say what the *function* of the cervix is – except to provide a useful sort of expandable entrance and exit to the womb.

Some women do derive considerable sexual pleasure from having it touched – particularly during the last 'surge' of intercourse – but others don't have any special feeling there.

This may be owing to individual variations in nerve supply to the cervix. Certainly, it's a remarkable fact that while many women feel *pain* when a surgical instrument has to be applied to the cervix, a whopping minority of the female population feel absolutely no painful sensation at all.

In this century, the cervix has developed one important new function – as a sort of useful hat-peg on which to hang a contraceptive cap. Any woman with a cap *must* be able to feel her cervix with her fingertips.

35

a disgrace – and now I'm afraid that the chickens are beginning to come home to roost.

Among the general shambles, a small number of women have not been told that their tests were positive. The odds against this happening are very long. But when it *does* happen, a woman may lose her life unnecessarily.

In the present confusion, my advice to all adult women is this. It's wildly unlikely that your doctor would fail to tell you that your smear test was positive. But just in case, you can protect yourself by asking for the result at your doctor's surgery or clinic, about six to eight weeks after having the test.

Disorders of the Cervix

CANCER OF THE CERVIX

Any woman (especially one who has not recently had a satisfactory smear) should watch out for the following symptoms:

Bleeding after intercourse

Bleeding between periods

Unexplained pain in the pelvic region, including pain on intercourse.

See your doctor within a few days, even if bleeding is confined to a few spots of blood or a faint brownish discharge. He should do an internal examination, look at the cervix and probably refer you to a gynaecologist – unless there's some obvious reason, such as that the contraceptive Pill you're taking doesn't suit you.

CERVICITIS. A form of inflammation which is quite common. The principal symptom is discharge. Simple local treatment as an outpatient is usually curative.

CERVICAL EROSION. This is a trivial complaint which can produce slight vaginal bleeding and discharge. It often occurs after childbirth. Treatment is hardly ever necessary unless an erosion produces pain on intercourse or a trying amount of discharge. In these cases, 'cautery' (with a chemical or hot or cold probe) should give a rapid and virtually painless cure.

POLYPS OF THE CERVIX. These occur at all ages, and cause discharge and slight bleeding. Removal is very easy.

Q I am worried about the possibility of getting cancer of the cervix. How can I find out when my next smear test is due?

A A simple way of finding out when your next smear is due is this:

In most parts of this country, your test will be recorded on a rectangular form, about the size of this page. The lab usually puts in the suggested date for your next smear on the form.

One copy of the form is sent to your GP, and one to whoever did the test (if it was done by someone other than your doctor).

At present, I'm afraid that the form is tending to take something like six to eight weeks to be returned to your doctor or clinic. So what you need to do is to contact your GP or clinic at the end of that time – and ask to be told the suggested date which has been written in on the form.

Q After reading many books and articles on the subject of cervical cancer, I find there's one question which still troubles me. As there now appears to be a great deal of evidence to show that the precursors of cancer of the cervix may be transmitted from the penis to the vagina, is there a danger of contracting carcinomas of the mouth or throat through oral sex?

A At the moment, there's no known relationship between oral love play and cancer of the mouth or throat. In fact oral or throat cancers are often closely linked with smoking – especially pipe-smoking – or with ill-fitting dentures rubbing on a sore place for many years.

Alcohol may play a part, and the oriental habit of chewing betel-nut is also said to be a factor in some cases. But often the cause isn't known. Mouth cancers actually seem to have become rarer during the course of this century, and standard surgical textbooks attribute this to the decline in clay pipe smoking.

In spite of the fact that there's now so much oral love play around, there's no suggestion that oral cancers are on the increase. But as with other forms of sex, it's very important to cut down all possible risks by being hygienic. No woman should do fellatio for a feller unless she's sure that he's clean and washed!

Q I am terrified about the prospect of getting cancer of the cervix. Is it true that there's some

birth control method that would protect me?

A Yes – both the sheath and
the diaphragm (cap) are thought to
give a woman some degree of
protection against cervical cancer.

Q My husband and I are in our
mid-50s, and have a won-
derful sex life, including oral sex. But
he is a heavy smoker, and I'm
worried that this could give me
cervical cancer.

A I don't think your husband's
smoking is likely to give you cervical cancer. The only known connection between the disease and
smoking is that it is more common
in smokers.

This may just be owing to two
factors:

Cancer of the cervix is much commoner down in socio-economic
groups IV and V (a fact which isn't
widely publicised, because people
are embarrassed about talking
about 'class' these days).

Smoking is *also* more common in
this section of the population.

There is no proof that smoking
causes cancer of the cervix. Unfortunately, there is now no doubt

whatever that smoking causes cancer of the lung (which kills 16 times
as many people as cancer of the

Protecting Yourself Against Cervical Cancer

In most western countries, cervical cancer kills nearly as many
women as road accidents do. But
in many poorer countries, the
death rate is much higher.

I cannot emphasise too
strongly that:

all women (except virgins) are
at risk

the disease is *preventable*.

We still don't really know why
cancer of the cervix occurs. It
certainly has a link with sex –
and this is the aspect that the
newspapers usually stress!

It's true that it only occurs in
women who have had sex – and
that it seems to be a bit more
common in women who have
had several lovers.

On the other hand, the newspapers rarely mention that this
appalling killer is also more
common in:

smokers

cervix), so I must be blunt and say that it's your husband – not you – who is in danger.

less well-off women

women who've had children

women over 35

women living in certain geographical areas.

But as I've said, *all* women who've ever had sex (even if it's only with their husbands) are liable to it. So unless you've led a totally celibate life (in which case, you're unlikely to be reading this book), *you owe it to yourself to take precautions against it.*

What precautions? Well first of all there's now considerable evidence that *barrier* methods of contraception (the cap or diaphragm, and the sheath) help protect a woman against cancer of the cervix.

Secondly, almost all doctors now agree that *all* adult women who have ever had sex should make sure they have regular smear tests.

In a smear test, all that happens is that the doctor uses a wooden spatula to scrape some cells off the cervix (the neck of the womb). The doctor puts these on a glass slide, and sends it to the laboratory for microscopic examination.

The point of the whole thing is this: *if there are any abnormal cells present, this gives very, very early warning of the disease – long before it causes any symptoms.* And at that stage, it's nearly always curable by laser therapy or a small biopsy ('sampling') operation.

Cancer of the cervix does eventually produce symptoms, but by the time it produces these symptoms, it's awfully late in the day. It's far, far better to detect it 10 or 20 years beforehand by the simple and – in most cases – painless technique of a smear test.

Q I'm very worried about the possibility of getting cancer of the cervix, because I have just realised that I am in one of the 'at risk' groups. This is because I had sex with a boy when I was a young teenager.

I am now 24, and the only other man I have slept with has been my husband.

A Then relax, ma'am. I keep trying to point out in this column that there are plenty of other 'risk factors' apart from having had teenage sex, for instance having dozens of lovers, being a manual worker, being a smoker.

And though cancer of the cervix can be awful if it's not 'caught' early, only one woman in 125 dies from this cause. The death figures for other tumours (such as cancer of the breasts or lungs) are far higher.

Also, I'd like to point out that at 24 time is very much on your side. Although the newspapers keep rabbiting on about 'epidemics' of cervical cancer in young women, you may be surprised to learn that the peak age for this disease is between 55 and 59!

I admit that there has been a worrying increase in cases in younger women lately. But if you have regular smear tests, the chance of you coming to any harm as a result of your teenage love affair is very, very small indeed.

Chlamydia

This is a 'new' infection, in the sense that it wasn't discovered all that long ago, and many people have never heard of it.

Yet millions of women worldwide have it – and in many cases it has affected their tubes and made them infertile. Regrettably, inexpensive tests for chlamydia aren't yet widely available (it doesn't show up on ordinary swabs). The result is that the condition often goes undiagnosed.

Chlamydia should be suspected if a woman has persistent vaginal/pelvic pain, with or without a fever and a discharge. Salpingitis (see below) may be present. It's vitally important to get treatment with the right antibiotic – penicillin is useless, but erythromycin or tetracycline usually work.

Circumcision

Circumcision remains popular in America, and in Jewish and Moslem cultures – but it's not very popular elsewhere. In Britain, less than 7% of all male babies are now circumcised – partly because of worries about the horrendous damage which can be done by a badly-performed circumcision (e.g. partial amputation of the penis).

However, circumcision does make it easier to keep the male organ clean, and so greatly cuts down on the risk of cancer of the penis in later life.

Most adults will have had the decision about circumcision taken for them by their parents. So the only point I want to make here is this: Dr Kinsey discovered that in many adult males, the foreskin will not 'go back' (or 'unpeel') when the penis is erect. That isn't a good state of affairs – either sexually or hygienically!

So if *your* foreskin is too tight to go back properly, then you owe it to yourself and your partner to see a doctor and have a circumcision done. Provided you consult an experienced surgeon, you should find this a relatively painless operation.

Q I feel abnormal, a freak, and a total failure as a woman. This is because of the fact I was born with a clitoris which is positioned outside my vagina. I've always felt that no man would ever find me attractive in bed because of this, so I've always turned them down.

Now I've fallen in love with the nicest man I've ever met. Yet I can't face the possibility of him rejecting me if he saw me naked.

Could I have an operation to make me normal? This is the most difficult letter I've ever written.

A Well, thank heavens you wrote! For I've got good news for you: the clitoris is *supposed* to be outside the vagina. It's tragic that you've spent so many years of unhappiness because of this mis-understanding about basic female anatomy.

A woman's clitoris is actually located well above the opening of her vagina, just in front of her pubic bone.

You desperately need some reassurance about your own anatomy. In your letter you say that you don't want to go to your own doc – so I suggest you get yourself examined by a woman medical officer at a family planning clinic. I'm sure she'll be very willing to check out your clitoris (and surrounding bits), and confirm that they're quite OK. Good luck.

Q I recently had a smear which was not quite right, so I went to a gynaecologist who did something called a 'colposcopy'.

He said everything was OK now, but can I trust him?

The Clitoris

From studying overseas editions of previous books of mine, I have been able to discover what the clitoris is called in various tongues. In German, it's *die Kitzler*, in Dutch it's *de clitoris*, in French it's *le cli-cli* – and in the Hebrew edition of one of my books it's represented by something that looks like the figures '72727', followed by a picture of Stonehenge!

The clitoris is located just in front of the pubic bone – so it will be gently compressed and squeezed during intercourse. It's only the size of a little button – even when it swells up during sexual excitement. Close examination of it reveals that it's in fact very similar in structure to a man's penis, so it's not surprising that it's more plentifully supplied with 'pleasure-producing' nerve endings than any other part of the female body.

Male readers may like to note that during love-play, many women (not all) do prefer to be stimulated along the *side* of the clitoris, rather than directly on top of it.

Disorders

Disorders of the clitoris are very rare. Occasionally, women seek medical advice because of a sudden and alarming *swelling* of the clitoris. This swelling appears to be due to a collection of blood – and it soon bursts, leaving no ill-effects.

Some years ago, I described the condition in *World Medicine*, and promptly received a number of letters from doctors who had also seen it. Two of them had discovered that their patients had actually caused the swelling by wrapping a cotton thread round the clitoris during masturbation – clearly, this is *not* a very sensible idea!

A Yup. A colposcopy is just like having your cervix examined by a very powerful pair of opera glasses. The great magnification gives the specialist an excellent idea of what's happening in the area where cancer is liable to develop.

The fact that you were able to get a colposcopy at all is *good* – many areas don't have this equipment. Be reassured; but keep on having smears at the intervals recommended by the doc.

Q I'm 45, and suddenly want to have a child for the first time. Is conception possible at this age? And if so, what are the possible risks which could affect the child?

A Yes, conception is usually possible in your 40s – though your fertility may well be much less than it was when you were in your 20s.

The main risk to the baby is that of Down's syndrome, which occurs with roughly this frequency:

Women under 30	1 in 1200
Women 40+	1 in 100
Women 45+	1 in 50

I hope you succeed in having a baby. Have fun trying.

Q Is it true that I will have more chance of having a baby if my husband dips his balls in very cold water immediately before we start to make love?

We have been trying for nearly a year, but have had absolutely no luck, so are willing to give anything a go.

A Well, as a general rule, men do produce more sperm if their testicles are cool.

That's why blokes with a low sperm count are usually advised to avoid getting over-heated – for instance, to steer clear of hot, nylon jockey-shorts, which raise the scrotal temperature to quite alarming heights!

It's true that some people have gone so far as to advise would-be fathers to increase their chances of conception by cooling down their wotsits.

The late, great Kenneth More popularised this technique on TV by talking about it when he and his wife were trying for a child.

But I'm afraid that dipping the testicles in icy water *just before making love* would be pointless (as well as being decidedly uncomfortable – for both of you!).

You see, sperm take many weeks to develop inside the testes. So 'ball-freezing' would have no effect on the sperm-count until about six weeks later.

If your man wants to dash out and sit in the December snow, that *might* improve his sperm count round about January or February. But it would be more sensible to go to an Infertility Clinic a.s.a.p. and try to find out *why* the pair of you have been having trouble conceiving.

Q Could the TB which I had many years ago be responsible for my current failure to conceive?

A Yes, possibly – TB can block the tubes. If you don't conceive fairly soon, seek help at an infertility clinic.

Q I am 24 years of age, married, and would love a baby – but after having tried for one for almost a year now, I am becoming rather worried. What should I do?

A If you've been trying for a year, then I think it's time to get some expert help.

Your GP may well be willing to do some initial tests (which I'll explain in a moment). If not, then try your local family planning clinic. If the initial tests don't reveal a cause for the difficulty in conceiving, then you and your husband will need to go to an infertility clinic for more sophisticated investigations. Initial tests include:

An internal examination of the woman

A brief physical check-up on the man

A sperm count on the man

A daily temperature chart kept by the woman for about six months –to try to see if she's ovulating

Possibly a post-coital test – in which the woman is examined internally soon after making love (to see how the sperms are getting on inside her)

Whichever doctor you see should also make some sort of inquiry to ensure that you're both 'doing it right'. Many couples aren't.

For instance, I recently came across a case in which a woman had undergone thousands of pounds' worth of time-consuming and uncomfortable investigations, which had shown she was perfectly normal. She had been too embarrassed to tell the specialist the real cause of the trouble – which was the fact that her husband couldn't get a good enough erection to get inside her.

Q I've just acquired an older lover. He says he needn't use a condom, as he couldn't possibly get anybody pregnant at his age.

But what is the oldest age at which a man has fathered a baby?

A 104. So unless your lover is at least 105 years old, he'd better 'don the con'!

Q Could I possibly get pregnant if my husband 'comes' outside me?

What worries me is that I might conceive if some sperm on a sheet got into my vagina.

A Just about possible, ma'am. A few cases of so-called 'virgin births' occur because the man's sperm gets deposited on a sheet or a thigh – and is transferred accidentally to the vagina (most often on the fingertips).

But once semen has dried out on a sheet, it's practically impossible for it to fertilise you.

Q I'm 35, and have an elderly 'boyfriend' of 71. Would a man of over 70 be able to father a child?

A Most definitely. Plenty of *over-80s* have done it – including Charlie Chaplin!

And in Elizabethan days, an old bloke called Thomas Parr got a poor serving wench with child at the age of 104 (him, not her).

Anyway, that was what she claimed – and he was probably too proud of himself to dispute it!

Q Is it possible for a woman to get pregnant if the man does not penetrate her, but simply comes outside?

A Yup. This is the explanation of a number of cases of alleged 'virgin birth' which have turned up in the Sunday newspapers over the years. (Some of them have been virgin on the ridiculous.)

Q Would the new contraceptive pill, called 'Dianette', help my spots and acne?

A Probably – but discuss it carefully with your doc first, as it's fairly powerful.

Condom

Although a lot of people are put off by the idea of the sheath, there is no doubt that it's one of the most popular and effective methods of contraception in the world. In most western countries, it's only just behind the Pill in the popularity stakes – and if there are any more Pill scares, it will probably regain the Number One position that it had in pre-Pill days.

I believe that more women should insist on their partners wearing a sheath – especially as, unlike the Pill or the IUD, it has virtually no side-effects. (A very few people are allergic to rubber, or to chemicals used in the process of vulcanization of rubber – but they can use 'hypo-allergenic' sheaths.)

There's also the very important plus-point that a sheath (like a diaphragm) probably helps to protect a woman against cancer of the cervix. It also gives at least some protection against any possible infection.

Indeed, sheaths are so useful that a small but increasing number of independent-minded women do carry them themselves for their own protection – and if they decide to go to bed with a lover, they make sure he uses one!

Some men who are having a bit of trouble with their potency do find it a little difficult to put a condom on – indeed, it's really quite common for women to say to a doctor, 'We can't use the sheath, because my husband can't get on with it . . .'

The answer to this problem is to make the putting on of the sheath *a part of love-play.* In other words, the woman can stimulate the man's penis with her hands until it's really hard. Then she can gently unroll the condom onto it. *That* usually solves the problem.

Note that sheath manufacturers have at last cottoned on to the

Q Is it true that there's some new French tablet that brings on your period each month, so you don't have to worry about using contraception?

A Yes, there is a French tablet called RU468, which does something rather like what you say. I have occasionally conversed on the phone – in broken French –

idea of making sheaths that will give women pleasure. They now make condoms with gentle 'ribbing' on the sides, so as to increase vaginal stimulation. Some women also appreciate the new coloured condoms, which look a lot better than the rather unattractive khaki shades of yesteryear.

Finally, it has to be admitted that sheaths do sometimes break. For that reason, many family planning specialists do recommend that you use a spermicide as an added precaution.

Some sheaths are now supplied with a pre-added spermicide. Alternatively, you can buy and use a *separate* spermicidal preparation. In Britain, it is common for a couple to insert a spermicidal pessary (vaginal tablet) about 10 minutes before intercourse: in America and some other countries, a spermicidal aerosol foam is more common.

with its inventor, Professor Etienne Baulieu, and he prefers to regard RU468 as 'an effective and safe method for termination of very early pregnancy' which can be used at the time the period is first noticed to be overdue.

But RU468 tends to cause heavy and prolonged bleeding, so it's not yet licensed for general use in Britain. If it is released in this country, there is bound to be a storm of moral outrage, because it could give every woman the power to abort herself each month if she wants to.

Q My wife and I have a very 'open' marriage, but of course I wouldn't like her to become pregnant by any of the other men she makes love with.

Our problem may strike you as silly, but we are too embarrassed to ask our doctor about it. Is it all right for her to use the same contraceptive 'cap' for each man? Or should she have a separate one for each person she sleeps with?

A There is no need for your wife to keep a separate cap for each bloke. Her life sounds quite complicated enough as it is, without having the additional problem of trying to remember which diaphragm she's supposed to be using.

But I think you and your wife should bear in mind that the cap does have a small failure rate – usually reckoned as about four pregnancies per 100 women per year.

If she does fall pregnant, you're certainly going to have a heck of a time working out who the father is.

Q I would really like to try that new contraceptive sponge you mentioned a long time ago in SHE. Is there any news of it being available in Britain yet?

A A lot of women are interested in the new vaginal sponge – probably for aesthetic reasons, because it isn't messy, and is a nice, 'feminine' thing to use.

It is now available over the counter in Britain, under the brand name 'Today'.

But here's the bad news. Attractive as this new method of contraception seems to be, the results of British trials have not been encouraging. In one test, no less than 25 out of 126 women became pregnant while using the sponge!

So I think that you should consider very carefully before deciding to rely completely on this new method for your protection.

Q I have recently had a mastectomy, because of breast cancer. This is enough to cope with on its own, but I find my main problem is with contraception. Having been advised to keep off the Pill

Cystitis

This means inflammation of the bladder, but in some cases which are labelled 'cystitis' there is inflammation of the rest of the urinary passages and even of the kidneys too. For this reason, cystitis is not entirely the trivial 'chill' that many people imagine it to be. In recent years, it has become clear that cystitis, unless properly treated, can sometimes have serious consequences on the kidneys.

The symptoms of cystitis are *pain on passing water* and *a frequent desire to do so*. There is sometimes a little blood in the urine. Quite often, these symptoms follow a woman's first experiences of love-making ('honeymoon cystitis').

As a general rule, cystitis is due to infection by germs which have entered the opening of the urinary passage (the urethra) and made their way up to the bladder.

In women, this passage is very, very short and, of course, very near the rectum – from which most such germs come. This is

(because I have had breast cancer) I went to a Family Planning Clinic to have a cap fitted.

However, as I am overweight, the doctor there said she couldn't fit either the cap or the coil because of the difficulty in finding my cervix!

So, am I to become resigned to

---

why cystitis is very common in women but very rare in men (except those with prostate trouble) – in fact, a man who developed cystitis without apparent reason would need a careful investigation of his urinary system, including X-rays, to see if some structural abnormality was present.

Treatment, if it's to be effective, has to be vigorous! It's certainly not sufficient to go along and ask the doctor for a bottle of medicine, and then forget about the whole thing if the symptoms go off in a couple of days.

Nowadays, the doctor will usually send a specially collected specimen of urine to the lab before he starts treatment – often a 10-day course of antibiotics. The result of this test will (with luck) let him know whether he's got you on the right antibiotic.

Incidentally, until the antibiotic starts working, you can relieve your pain by drinking plenty of liquid, putting a hot-water bottle over your bladder, and taking a little bicarbonate of soda.

However, the world-famous 'Kilmartin self-help regime' says that you should also:

avoid bubble baths and all other possible chemical irritants

wash your genital area daily with a clean cloth which you boil after use – and keep for no other purpose

in the event of an attack of cystitis, take a painkiller

then drink plenty of water with a level teaspoon of bicarbonate of soda

finally, apply one hot-water bottle to your lower abdomen, and place another one between your thighs.

Remember too that as cystitis is so very often started off by love-play or love-making (and especially by *inept* efforts at love-play), it's a good idea to insist that your partner is gentle, careful and clean when he handles this delicate area of your body.

using sheaths? This must be a common problem for 'mastectomees', since we are told that we should not become pregnant for five years after having breast cancer.

A Yes, this is indeed a common problem, ma'am – and thank you for your very jolly and cheerful letter, which must have been written in the face of some adversity (to put it mildly).

Roughly one woman in every 15 develops breast cancer, and most of those who have the misfortune to get it do have some form of mastectomy operation.

Since breast cancer is usually a 'hormone-dependent' growth, it's true that (as you say) most patients are advised not to use the Pill afterwards. For the same reasons, most women are advised by their surgeons not to become pregnant for some years after having the cancer removed.

So what are all these thousands of women going to use for birth control after the operation? For it's important to realise that most of them are, like yourself, interested in sex – and sexually attractive – despite having been ill.

The basic choices left are:

1 the sheath;
2 the coil (IUD);
3 the cap (diaphragm);

4 the new chemical sponge (which will be available by the time this appears in print);
5 vasectomy;
6 female sterilisation;
7 some variation of the rhythm method ('safe period').

I *haven't* included either the mini-Pill (progestogen-only Pill) or 'the shot' (the contraceptive injection), because there are considerable doubts as to whether they should be given to women who've had breast cancer.

If you don't want to have any more children, then you and your husband should seriously consider vasectomy or female sterilisation. But if you *do* want more babies, the choice lies between methods 1, 2, 3, 4 and 7. With all due respect to the doctor who has examined you, I don't think that method 2 (the coil) and method 3 (the cap) are necessarily ruled out because of the difficulty in finding your cervix.

Certainly, you can't use a cap till somebody has taught you to find your own cervix. But a doctor who is very experienced in IUD work ought to be able to find your cervix and insert a coil for you. Ask your own GP for the name of someone in your area who is practised in difficult IUD insertions.
Good luck.

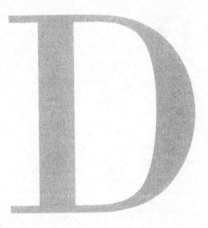

Q From the moment I first had sex, I have been plagued with cystitis. Each act of intercourse makes it worse, and my GP seems to be unable to do anything about it.

A Discuss with him or her whether the time has now come for a referral to a urologist.

Q I see that you have had a lot of letters from cystitis sufferers. I don't know whether you think this would help, but I found that both myself and my daughter were cured of cystitis when we stopped eating pears. Do you think that cystitis could be due to an allergy to pears?

A I don't know – but certainly food sensitivities now seem to be much more common than was previously thought. So cystitis sufferers might like to try avoiding pears, and see what happens. Incidentally, some women with cystitis seem to do better if they avoid alcohol.

Q What exactly is a 'D and C'? My doctor said I needed one, and has given me a letter to take to a surgeon to have it done.

But when I asked him what it was, he just laughed and said it was 'a sort of de-coke of the engine'.

A Um, yes – us male docs do

Diet

Yes – diet and your sex life are linked! If you let your body become obese and out of shape, you'll probably damage your sex life.

Also, good nutrition does seem to have a beneficial effect on most human activities – and it seems highly probable that it's good for sexual activity too. At present, the best medical opinion is that if you want a good all-round diet, you should eat plenty of the following:

green vegetables (including peas, beans, lettuce, cabbage, cauliflower and spinach)

root vegetables (carrots, turnips, swede and potatoes – yes, potatoes!)

fish

wholemeal bread

fruit

Despite what manufacturers

say, you should try and steer clear of too much:

salt

butter

cheese

fried food

fatty meats

cream

anything that contains saturated (mainly animal) fats – including pastry and cookies

alcohol – especially spirits.

It's a bit hard to say whether *sugar* should be added to this list. Certainly, sugar is nowhere near as fattening as most people imagine – but it does provide 'empty' calories (which seem to be of no real nutritional value).

Also – despite the understandable efforts of the sugar industry to convince us otherwise – it

tend to make unfortunate remarks like that. Anyway, let me try to explain it a bit more fully. A D and C is the commonest operation performed in this country, with about 140,000 women undergoing the procedure each year. The initials stand for 'dilatation and curettage' – and what *that* means is: widening the channel through the neck of the womb so that an instrument can be passed through it; using the aforesaid instrument to curette – scrape out – the lining of the womb. A D and C is very often known simply as 'a scrape'.

It can be useful as a means of diagnosing womb disorders, because it enables surgeons to take out pieces of womb lining and examine them under the microscope.

Also, it can be an effective form of treatment (as opposed to diagnosis) for some womb conditions. For example, a D and C is an efficient way of removing pieces of afterbirth (placenta), which are often left behind after childbirth or miscarriage.

In Britain, the procedure is almost invariably done under general anaesthetic, so it should be painless. And it's done through your vagina, so there's no cutting of the skin. On the other hand, there is now some feeling that too many D and Cs are being done. By my calculation, very nearly half the women in Britain will end up having one – which does seem a bit excessive, to put it mildly!

So talk the operation over carefully with the surgeon, and make sure that it's necessary before you go ahead.

does rot your teeth!

Of course, nearly all of us enjoy a good meal of 'forbidden' foods now and again. And there's no doubt that a thoroughly wicked meal – with all the things you're not really supposed to eat – can be the prelude to a highly successful evening in bed.

Perhaps I should add that if you believe in *aphrodisiac* foods, then there's no harm at all in adding them to your diet. I have to say, however, that there's no medical evidence that champagne, oysters, *coquilles St. Jacques* or octopus actually work.

But the good thing about allegedly aphrodisiac foods is that if a person *believes* in them, then they'll do her or him some good. Also, if your dinner partner orders oysters and champagne, you do at least have some idea of what she or he has in mind!

Dyspareunia

'Ye Gods,' I hear you say, 'What's dyspareunia? (And how do you pronounce it?)'

Well, it's pronounced 'diss-par-YEW-nya'. And it means 'pain on intercourse'. For some reason, the term dyspareunia is almost always applied to pain experienced by women.

Now, what can cause pain during intercourse?

The first group of physical causes are the common (all too common!) vaginal infections. These are: thrush (candida); trichomonas ('trich'); certain other infections, and, occasionally, herpes.

Clearly, the remedy for all these is to get yourself (and, if necessary, your partner) diagnosed and treated as soon as possible. (If you don't want to see your GP, you can call your local health authority for the address of your nearest Special Clinic.) Your local Well-Woman Clinic may also be able to help,

although not all of them are able to prescribe treatment.

Non-infectious causes of intercourse pain include the following:

Urethral caruncle: a swelling occurring at the opening of the waterworks. Treatment: removal.

Endometriosis: an inflammatory condition of the internal organs; tends to cause *deep* pain on sex. Treatment: hormones or surgery.

Post-menopause vaginitis: tenderness caused by the drop in female hormones. Treatment: female hormones.

Post-episiotomy (or post-childbirth tear) pain: Lubricants such as KY, Durol or Senselle may help. If not, see a gynae expert.

Prolapsed ovary: if your ovary is lying too low in your pelvis, this can cause pain in some positions of intercourse. Treatment: choose another position.

Cervical erosion: at least one in ten women has an erosion of the

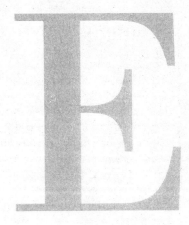

cervix. This may occasionally cause deep dyspareunia. Treatment: usually cautery of the erosion.

Uncommonly in Britain, deep pain may be due to the chronic disability called pelvic inflammatory disease (PID). Very, very rarely, it may be due to cancer of the cervix.

Note that I have not listed a 'small vagina' as a physical cause of intercourse pain. Though many people still believe in the myth of the small vagina as a common reason for pain, I've not seen a single case since I qualified in 1962.

In fact, nearly all alleged cases of 'narrow vagina' turn out to be due to a fantastically common emotional problem called vaginismus, in which the pelvic muscles tighten up whenever an approach is made to the vagina. This can usually be cured or helped by relaxation therapy.

ECTOPIC PREGNANCY

Ectopic Pregnancy

This means pregnancy occurring outside the normal situation (i.e. the womb). In the great majority of such cases, the fertilised egg lodges in the Fallopian tube (which connects the ovary to the womb). Where this happens there is virtually no possibility that the baby can be born.

In fact, it usually becomes apparent that something is wrong not long after the first period is missed. The symptoms vary a good deal, but usually the woman experiences quite severe pain low down in the abdomen, on either the right or the left side, depending on which tube is involved. Sometimes the pain is accompanied by giddiness. Within a few hours there is usually vaginal bleeding.

In some cases of ectopic pregnancy there is severe bleeding inside the abdomen. If this happens, the patient collapses and is pale, shocked and gasping for breath. She *must* be got to hospital immediately.

The only treatment for ectopic pregnancy is to remove the foetus by surgical operation. Usually the Fallopian tube has to be taken away as well. This doesn't mean that the patient is now sterile, however; if the other tube is healthy, there is no reason why she should not have children in the future.

Ectopic pregnancies are probably commoner in women who are using the IUD – and possibly in women who are on the mini-Pill.

Q May I give a word of encouragement to your reader who wondered if she could have a baby after having an ectopic pregnancy? I had an ectopic, and was therefore left with only one tube. But afterwards, I was lucky enough to produce three children.

A Thank you very much, ma'am! Good of you to give this encouragement to the many women who've had ectopics.

Q I've had an ectopic pregnancy; as a result, one of my tubes was removed. We've been trying since then to start a family, but no luck. What are my chances?

56

A Perfectly all right – *if* your other tube is OK. If you've been trying unsuccessfully for over a year, then I think it's time you went to a gynaecologist to have a test to reveal whether this tube is bunged up or not.

Good luck.

Exercise

There's no doubt that sensible exercise benefits your general health. For that reason, a sensible amount of exercise is likely to benefit your sex life too – simply by toning up your body.

The widespread belief that exercise – and, in particular, jogging – will reduce your libido is nonsense! I keep encountering athletes who assure me that 'medical research' has proved that running makes you less sexy.

Well, the 'medical research' in question was an April Fool's Day joke published by my own medical journal, *General Practitioner*! We ran a completely bogus story – made up by a Buckinghamshire GP, Dr Bev Daily – about how a completely fictional American university had shown that exercise makes people lose their interest in sex because it raises the temperature in their running shorts!

This wonderfully daft story was swallowed hook, line and sinker by the London *Daily Mail*, and was duly published and flashed round the world. All our subsequent efforts to convince people that the story was a hoax have failed, and it's still quoted. If they were to look at the original article, they'd find that the giveaway was a small paragraph near the end in which Dr Daily claimed that scientists were even now working on a device to combat 'exercise-induced loss of libido' – a pocket refrigerator to be worn inside the shorts!

In all this, however, there is one faint echo of truth. It's this: really *intensive* exercise over a long spell of time (the sort of thing that serious Olympic contenders engage in) does have an effect on women's sex glands – it takes their periods away. Indeed, I am reliably informed that the highly-trained women's athletics squads of most western nations have almost all of them lost their periods at one time or another.

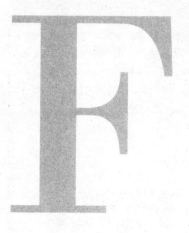

The Fallopian Tubes

Your 'tubes' are among the most vital organs of your body – vital to the human race that is. Why? Because until very recently, it was completely impossible for a baby to be born unless his or her mum had at least one healthy fallopian tube. And unfortunately, women's tubes are often far from healthy.

Fallopian tubes are the little bits of tubing which link your ovaries to your womb. You have a left tube and a right tube. Each one is about 4" (10cm) long. The outer end makes a sort of funnel shape which points towards your ovary, the idea being that when an egg is released from the ovary, it'll go into the funnel and find its way down the tube and into your womb.

It's thought that fertilisation usually takes place within the tube – in other words, that's where the sperm meets the egg. And once the egg's been fertilised, it tries to find a suitable place on the womb lining on which to implant.

The *inside* of the tube is extremely narrow, and it's lined with cells which project out into the tube like stalactites and stalagmites in a long, narrow cave.

Blocked Tubes

A tremendously common cause of infertility in women is blocked tubes. If the Fallopian tubes are blocked for any reason, the man's sperm can't get through to the woman's ova.

The causes of this difficulty are:

a previous sterilization operation (some women undergo sterilization, then get divorced and remarried and want their tubes unblocked)

previous infection of the tubes;

inflammatory disorders in the lower abdomen – for instance, reaction to a past burst appendix, or endometriosis.

I have to say that tube blockage due to previous infection of the tubes is far more common than most people realise, and that these infections are often – though very far from always – sexually transmitted.

However, your tubes *can* become infected in other ways, for instance, as a result of using an IUD. I'm not suggesting that if you have blocked tubes, you should feel guilty about some affair of long ago.

How Do You Find Out Your Tubes Are Blocked?

If you have had serious difficulties in conceiving, then the infertility experts will usually want to investigate you for possible tube blockage. This *can't* be diagnosed by a simple vaginal examination. It has to be done by one of these means:

special X-rays of the tubes

injecting gas through the tubes to see if it goes through freely

laparoscopy.

How To Get Treated

Firstly, it may sometimes be possible to treat the underlying disease – for instance, if an infection is still present, to treat it with antibiotics. The common cause of tube blockage, endometriosis, can often be successfully treated with hormones or surgery (including laser surgery).

Secondly, a totally blocked tube can sometimes be repaired by delicate surgery, working with an operating microscope (microsurgery).

Thirdly, the 'test-tube baby' technique may be used to bypass the blockage altogether.

Fertilisation

I find it incredible that each of us is here because a single microscopic sperm met a single microscopic ovum in somebody's Fallopian tube. Or – in the case of test-tube babies – in somebody's laboratory.

That is, of course, what 'fertilisation' means – the union of a man's sperm with a woman's ovum (egg).

What happens is that when a couple make love, a living pool of sperm is deposited around the woman's cervix. It usually contains anything between 300 million and 500 million of the little 'tadpoles'.

Most of the fluid eventually runs out of the vagina. But a large number of the sperms streak upwards, through the cervix, through the womb, and into the Fallopian tubes, looking for a likely ovum to fertilise.

If the woman has just ovulated (this tends to happen at mid-cycle), just such an ovum will be innocently making its way down one of the Fallopian tubes.

The fastest and most determined of the sperms reaches her, penetrates her – and that's that! Some might say that there's an interesting analogy with male human behaviour here . . .

Fertilisation usually seems to take place in the outer third of a woman's Fallopian tube, but it could occur either higher up or lower down.

Unfortunately, if it occurs *too* high up (before the ovum has actually got into the funnel-like opening of the Fallopian tube) the result will probably be an ectopic – i.e. 'out of place' – pregnancy. This can hardly ever survive.

And if fertilisation occurs too low down (for instance, if the sperm and ovum meet in the womb) then again there's no chance that the fertilised ovum will live.

But if the woman and man have synchronised their love-making correctly so that the ripe ovum and the intrepid sperm meet in the right place, then the two of them will fuse together – and the resulting fertilised ovum will continue on its passage down the Fallopian tube and into the womb, where with luck it will 'implant' in the womb lining a few days later.

In practice, it does seem that a very high percentage of fertilised ova fail to implant in the lining of the womb. In these cases, the woman simply menstruates – and never even realises that her ovum was fertilised that month.

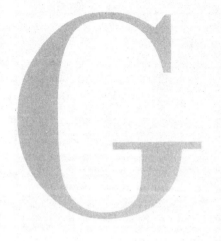

Gardnerella

This is a relatively newly discovered vaginal infection, but one
which is increasingly commonly
diagnosed, especially in the
USA.

The chief symptom is a
greyish vaginal discharge.
Response to the drug metronidazole is good.

Gonorrhoea

This form of VD is regrettably
still common in every country in
the world. In men, gonorrhoea
produces two dramatic symptoms, about two to five days
after having sex with someone
who is infected. These are:
severe pain on passing water
('like passing razor blades'),
and a copious discharge from
the penis.

There can be other symptoms
if you've taken part in oral or
other forms of sex. And there
can be very serious and painful
complications later.

Fortunately, treatment with
adequate doses of penicillin
cures most people. But at all
costs, don't sleep with anyone
till you're cured. This kind of
behaviour is almost criminally

stupid – yet some men are thoughtless enough to do it.

The most tragic thing about gonorrhoea is that *in most women it produces no symptoms.* In some instances, there may be an episode of pain, fever or vaginal discharge. But in most cases, what happens is that the woman makes love with somebody (perhaps someone she has a holiday romance with), becomes infected, but *doesn't realise.*

For months or even years thereafter, the gonorrhoea germ may be damaging her health – and specifically the health of her pelvic organs. It may make her sterile, or give her salpingitis.

Fortunately, many women *do* have their cases diagnosed – because the infection is detected in their partner and he tells them that they need treatment.

So, if you ever feel that you have 'taken a risk' get a full confidential check-up – preferably at a specialist Genito-Urinary Clinic of the type available in Britain and some other countries.

Once gonorrhoea has been successfully diagnosed it can be treated – usually very successfully, if it's caught early enough. Treatment is usually with penicillin.

Penicillin-resistant gonorrhoea can usually be defeated by other drugs, such as spectinomycin.

Finally, here are a few tips for avoiding gonorrhoea and other types of VD:

avoid casual sex and one-night stands

consider using a barrier method of contraception – it helps a bit

be wary of dates with men who are air travellers – international travellers have been shown to be particularly liable to acquire and spread VD (often the resistant kind)

if in doubt after a sexual contact, always have an internal check-up.

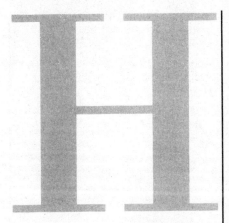

Q I would kill myself if it weren't for the fact that I have a child to support. After 15 years of faithful but not very happy marriage, I separated from my husband last year.

For a while after that I had the most fantastic time. I hadn't realised that men would find me so attractive. I had four lovers in a row — and sex with them was wonderful (far better than it was with my husband). It was beautiful to find that I could go on for hours and hours. I was very happy.

Then it happened: I got herpes. I understand that there is nothing that can be done, and that I can never make love again.

A No, that isn't true. I happen to know the very well-qualified doctor who is treating you, and if you go and see him again he will tell you (a) that herpes often does burn itself out; (b) that new drugs are giving promising results; and (c) that a cure will probably be found eventually. Good luck.

Q I am faithful to my boyfriend, and he has been faithful to me.

But four months ago, I developed small blisters at the opening of my vagina. The clinic was very nice, but told me it was herpes.

I felt so ashamed that I never mentioned it to anyone, not even my boyfriend.

But as the attack of herpes was really very mild, is there a chance it won't come back?

A Yes, this is possible. But the odds are that you may get further attacks. If so, let's hope they're mild ones again.

What worries me is that you haven't told your boyfriend! Presumably you acquired the herpes virus from him – or perhaps you got it from a previous lover. If the latter is true, then you may have infected your boyfriend too.

So I feel the most honest thing to do would be to tell him the truth – and to go back together to the Genito-Urinary Clinic ('Special Clinic') for mutual counselling.

Q Sometimes my fiancé develops minute blister-like lesions on his penis. And I sometimes experience a severe burning sensation after passing water. Could this be serious?

A I have to be frank and say that there's a chance this could be herpes. (But as I've said before,

herpes isn't as big a reason for panic as the newspapers seem to think.)

Anyway, both of you should definitely go to a 'special clinic' for a confidential check-up.

Q Is it true that there's some sort of organisation for people who have had herpes?

A Yes, write to the Herpes Association c/o *Spare Rib, 27 Clerkenwell Close, London EC1 0AT.*

Q I have definitely contracted vaginal herpes as a direct result of having oral sex when my partner had a cold sore on his mouth.

I feel strongly that you should immediately advise everybody not to participate in oral sex while suffering from an outbreak of cold sores.

A I do agree. In fact, I have long advised against having oral love play whilst people are suffering from *any* kind of mouth or throat infection.

The virus which causes the common 'cold sore' on the lip is so similar to the virus of genital herpes that it may eventually transpire that the current outbreak of genital herpes in the USA and Britain is linked with the fact that oral sex has become so popular in the last two decades or so.

I'm sorry to hear about your herpes, and hope you succeed in defeating it.

Q
I am getting very bad menopause symptoms. Would hormone therapy be the answer?

A
Hormone replacement therapy (HRT) helps most women with

Herpes

So many people are worried about herpes; however, the statistical chance of catching it in Britain (in contrast to the USA) is still low, with only about 12,000 reported cases a year.

But everybody ought to know the classic symptoms. These include painful little blisters on the sex organs – rather like the 'cold sores' so many people get on their mouths. (In fact, the virus which causes cold sores is very closely related to the one which causes herpes.) There can be many other symptoms, including itching, inability to pass water, fever, headache and muscle pains. But it's the blisters you should look out for.

If you think you've got herpes, you should get yourself to a *Sexually Transmitted Disease clinic*

as fast as possible. There's still no actual cure for the infection, but the drug acyclovir (Zovirax) relieves symptoms and reduces the duration of attacks. There is a vaccine, but it doesn't seem to work. Press reports of a 'cure' invented by 'Dr' Stephan (of the so-called 'Harley St Hit-Man' case) are nonsense: Mr Stephan isn't really a doctor, and does not have a cure for herpes.

But let me finish with one piece of relatively good news. Most members of the public seem to be convinced that 'Herpes is forever'. This is now known to be untrue. Many people only have one single attack, and there is a definite tendency for the disease to burn itself out. So if you've got herpes, please *don't* despair.

menopause symptoms – but nothing is 100% certain in medicine, and I can't promise that you'd be helped.

However, if I were a woman with severe 'change of life' symptoms I think that I'd unhesitatingly take the hormones for a spell – provided that they were given under careful supervision, with regular health checks. Good luck.

Q I'm a woman of 47 and I am really desperate because the hormone treatment which I'm having for the menopause isn't helping my appalling baldness. I am even losing possible jobs because of my appearance. NHS wigs look awful and I'm short of money for a top-class one.

A I'm sorry to hear about this. You are seeing one of the most famous endocrinologists in the country, and you should ask him whether there is any hope at all that the baldness will get better. If the answer's 'no' then I think you could try one of the following: a good class wig, a hair transplant, or hair 'weaving'. I'm afraid all of these are very expensive. But since your baldness is having such a disastrous effect on your employment prospects, I'm sure that any bank manager would be willing to give

you a long-term loan to cover the cost. Good luck.

Q I have just reached the menopause, and my doctor has put me on hormone replacement therapy for hot flushes. What I want to know is, do I need to go on

Hygiene

First things first. How do you keep the intimate, sexual places of your body in the best possible trim?

Whether you are a man or a woman, a daily wash of the genital organs in hand-hot water with mild soap is a must. You don't actually need to have a bath every day of your life, though of course many people find it invigorating and refreshing.

Too *many* baths can in fact be bad for the sex organs. Many women, and some men, find that they keep getting irritating attacks of thrush and other fungus infections if they have too many hot baths. If *you* have any tendency to thrush or to those trying fungal infections of the skin between the thighs, you would almost certainly do better to have cool showers than hot tubs.

taking it for the rest of my life?

I feel that if I don't go on taking it, by the time I'm 55, I'll be looking like Phil Collins instead of Joan Collins!

A You will need it until you find that when you have a break, the hot flushes don't come back. But you can take it for longer (indeed, for ten or 20 years), if your doc agrees, and if you feel it's doing you good.

There are risks from 'HRT', but some gynaecologists now think women should take it for life to avoid osteoporosis (brittle bone disease).

Whether you are female or male, *avoid* applying chemical agents to your genital area. Be especially wary if you have sensitive skin or are prone to allergic reactions. Even bubble baths can sometimes be harmful to those delicate tissues!

Because men's genitals are less complicated, they have less to worry about where health and hygiene are concerned. However, a man *does* have to keep his genitals in reasonable hygienic trim, for three reasons:

if you don't observe the simple rules of hygiene described below, you increase your chances of cancer of the penis.

men who aren't hygienic tend to give their sexual partners certain illnesses – including, possibly, cancer of the cervix

unless you keep yourself clean 'down below', you're likely to discover that women find you, to say the least, unappealing, especially where oral sex is concerned!

Some readers may find it incredible that it's necessary to tell the above facts to any man. But I do assure you that doctors find that a distressing proportion of the men whom they have to examine have simply *no* idea of personal genital hygiene at all. (Yuk!)

All males should wash their genitals at least once a day, paying special attention to the part of the male organ just below the 'head' – this is where the skin glands produce a material called 'smegma', which rapidly accumulates in unhygienic males.

If the man isn't circumcised, he should take care to draw his foreskin back before washing.

Hysterectomy

An incredible one in five of all women have this operation at some stage in their lives, so it's well worth your while knowing exactly what it involves. Hysterectomy just means removal of the womb or uterus, and nothing else.

Because few people understand anatomy, they tend to get confused about hysterectomy in two ways. Firstly, they often think that the operation involves taking away all or part of the vagina and will therefore make it impossible for the woman to have intercourse ever again. This is nonsense.

No part of the vagina is removed. When the womb has been taken out, this leaves a little gap at the very top of the vagina, and that gap is sewn up by the surgeon.

Some gynaecologists say that this actually makes the vagina a bit longer than it was before. Anyway, it certainly isn't any smaller, so it'll be just as effective a love-making organ as ever it was. Once the stitches at the very top of the vagina have healed, you'll be able to resume love-making just as before.

Some women find that their climaxes feel a little different because the womb has gone. Many women enjoy sex more than they did before for two reasons: whatever womb condition they were suffering from has been cured, and now that the womb has been removed, the fear of unwanted pregnancy is gone forever.

A second source of confusion is the muddle in people's minds over the womb and the ovaries. Many women (and men) think that if you have a hysterectomy this will stop your output of female hormones: they believe that you will therefore get hot flushes, put on weight, become neurotic and goodness only knows what else besides. Once again, this is utter nonsense. It is the ovaries, not the womb, which produce female hormones. *As long as the ovaries aren't removed at the same time*, your hysterectomy won't produce any of the distressing symptoms of hormone deficiency.

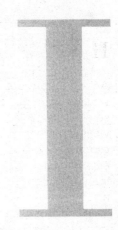

Removal of the Ovaries

Regrettably, it is sometimes necessary to remove the ovaries at the same time as a hysterectomy is done, though this only happens in a minority of cases. The ovaries may have to be taken out because they contain cysts or because they're diseased.

If the surgeon removes them while you're still young (indeed, at any stage before the change of life), then I'm afraid that there's every chance that the resulting sharp drop in hormones will give you quite severe menopausal symptoms in the days after the operation – mainly in the form of hot flushes and sweating attacks. There may also be vaginal dryness later on.

Fortunately, however, these distressing symptoms can be prevented with carefully prescribed doses of female hormones over the next few months or even years. But make sure you get the treatment: a disquieting number of younger women complain that they were never offered it.

Implantation

What is implantation? Well, it's the process whereby a fertilised egg (ovum) becomes embedded in your womb.

Fertilisation – which is the union of a sperm with your ovum – normally takes place in the outer part of one of your Fallopian tubes.

But that doesn't necessarily mean that you're going to get pregnant. The fertilised ovum has quite a way to go before it embeds itself in your womb lining and starts to put down roots into it. That's implantation.

The fertilised ovum is impossible to see with the naked eye. It makes its way through the long cavern of your Fallopian tube, emerges into the uterus, and then may or may not find a suitable spot on the womb lining in which to embed itself.

If it doesn't find a suitable spot, then that particular ovum will be lost – and you won't become pregnant that month. This often happens.

The journey from the point of fertilisation down to the point of implantation takes quite a time – it's thought to be five to seven days in most cases. Implantation doesn't occur till nearly a week after you made love.

That time gap of five to seven days is of tremendous practical and philosophical importance these days. Why? Because it's on that time gap that the whole principle of the 'Morning After Pill' and the 'Morning After Coil' is based.

You see, many doctors now feel that it is not wrong to pre-

Q I notice you often recommend Family Planning Clinics as a source of help for sex problems. I took my impotent husband to one near us, but they didn't want to know.

A Oh dear. Not all Family Planning Clinics provide 'Balint treatment' – a form of brief psychotherapy/counselling which helps many men and women with sex problems. The cuts of recent years have had a disastrous effect on clinic services in many areas.

So here are two alternative sources of help and counselling for your husband. Send a large s.a.e., to either of these two organisations, asking for the name of their nearest available therapists to: The

vent pregnancy by giving a special pill (or fitting an IUD) between the time of fertilisation and the time of implantation.

Others feel that it *is* wrong, and that to do it is to take life.

Certainly, the fertilised ovum is living (as, indeed, are the sperms and the unfertilised ovum). But a world authority on conception and contraception, Dr John Guillebaud says that as a Christian doctor he feels that pregnancy is not established till implantation has taken place – and that therefore it is not immoral to prevent that implantation.

The philosophical issues are very complex. But the law certainly makes no objection to the use of 'Morning-After' methods in order to prevent implantation.

Institute of Psycho-Sexual Medicine, *11 Chandos Street, London W1M 9DE*; The Association of Sexual and Marital Therapists, *PO Box 62, Sheffield S10 3TS.* Good luck.

Q In our 31-year marriage my husband has had intercourse with me exactly three times. I have spent my married life crying myself to sleep because of this. But we have never, ever discussed it. Only now (when I have reached the menopause) have I broken down in tears in front of him. But I suppose it's too late to do anything now?

A Not necessarily, ma'am. Your long and sad letter suggests that your husband has a considerable impotence problem. But if your GP sent the pair of you to a sex therapist, it could be sorted out.

And even if it couldn't, the therapist could still guide you both to loving and gentle ways of obtaining mutual fulfilment. Good luck to you.

Impotence

The American sex researchers, Masters and Johnson claimed impotence to affect 40% of American marriages to some extent, and the same *might* possibly be true of other countries, though figures are lacking. Certainly, the problem's a very widespread one.

Many cases of impotence are thought by doctors to be psychological in origin. Among the exceptions are impotence associated with diabetes and blood-vessel disease, and impotence caused by drugs, *e.g.* tablets for high blood pressure, and alcohol.

Most patients find difficulty in accepting that their problems could be due to stress, tiredness or emotional hang-ups, and willingly ascribe their impotence to such improbable causes as hormone or vitamin deficiency, or to advancing age. They may fall into the clutches of quacks, and spend a good deal of money on useless but expensive 'tonics', 'rejuvenatives', and 'aphrodisiacs'.

Unfortunately, the impotent patient who goes to his doctor may not always obtain a great deal of help, for several reasons. In the first place, as a medical journal grimly remarked recently, 'the doctor may be in the same boat himself'. Regrettably, a doctor's training doesn't usually include much formal teaching on sexual problems, and it is unfortunately true that many middle-aged men are erroneously told that their impotence is due to their age. In fact, age is no bar to sexual performance: many men are quite potent at 80 or even 90!

There is no short and easy answer to the problem of impotence. Patients will often demand hormone tablets or injections from their doctors, before eventually discovering that no magic 'instant remedy' exists.

What *can* be done about impotence then? Where there's no *physical* cause, the patient and his partner should learn to accept the fact that his problem

Q My mother, aged 77, is very fit and still rides a bike. But her problem is that she is often very incontinent of urine. I suppose it's old and weak muscles, is it?

A Yes, it's a similar problem to the 'lax pelvic floor' one. But your mum's symptoms are so severe that she really ought to consult a gynaecologist – to see whether a 'tightening-up' op is what's needed.

Q I am a nurse, and pregnant. I know that my husband's seminal fluid contains prostaglandins, and remember learning that these can induce labour. Could I use

is an understandable emotional one. When this is done, and he recognises that he is not suffering from either some horrible disease or from 'lack of manhood', the problem is then cut down to size and becomes simply a matter of overcoming his own sexual repressions and anxieties or tiredness!

A surprising number of men will achieve this victory over a period of time, sometimes aided by rest, a change of job, or anti-depressants. For others, however, recovery may be very difficult, even with the help of a loving and understanding wife. A 'second honeymoon' together, away from children and the stress of work, may be of considerable value.

The most effective therapy available is the 'sexual retraining' developed in the USA by Masters and Johnson. But in Britain the impotent man and his wife will derive very considerable benefits from learning similar techniques to those of Masters and Johnson taught at many National Marriage Guidance Council centres ('Relate') and Family Planning Clinics.

Happily, the last few years have seen major improvements in the treatment of the type of impotence that is due to physical causes. Urological surgeons can now insert 'splints' (including inflatable splints) into the penis. They can also prescribe injections, which can be given directly into the penis in order to produce an immediate erection.

sex as a way of starting labour?

Also, when I reach a climax during pregnancy, what effect does it have on the baby?

A Remarkably little research has been done on the effect of maternal climax during pregnancy. I know of no evidence that it does the baby any harm.

Male sex fluid does contain the chemicals called prostaglandins, and these compounds can induce labour (knowledge based on the discovery of the rather yukky practice of a remote African tribe – who use an *oral* draught of semen to induce labour).

I'm open to correction, but I doubt whether having ordinary intercourse would deliver enough prostaglandins to the area of the uterus to make you go into labour.

Q My doctor has recommended a coil for me. But I'm not married, and I thought that it was contra-indicated for single women?

A Well, the intra-uterine device (IUD) is fine for most women *who have had children.*

The smaller types of IUD can easily be fitted in women who've never been pregnant. But the risk of side-effects (such as infection) does seem to be quite high – particularly if the person has several lovers.

I do not say that you *mustn't* have an IUD. But I do reckon you should get a second opinion from a Family Planning Clinic first.

Q I am 21 and have only recently starting having sex. Would the IUD be a good method for me to choose, as one of my friends has suggested?

A Doctors are now increasingly wary about fitting intra- uterine devices into 'nullips' – that is, women who've never been pregnant.

This is mainly because the risks of pelvic infection seem to be considerably higher in this group. No one knows why this should be. But it's been suggested that one factor may be that single women tend to have multiple partners.

Pelvic infection can have disastrous effects on your health and fertility. (For instance, it may block your tubes.) So think very carefully indeed before you agree to have an IUD.

Q I have had a coil for some time, and it was fine to begin with. But suddenly I've starting having periods that are two weeks long. Why?

A It's normal for periods to be longer on the coil and other types of IUD – but not as long as this.

When a woman who's using an IUD suddenly starts getting very long or painful periods, there must be some cause. *Very often, the device has started to come out.*

So get yourself a check-up from a GP or family planning clinic soonest – meantime, avoid sex as you may be at risk of pregnancy if the coil is coming out.

Q I am 23 and have just lost my virginity. Would you recommend that I use the IUD as a contraceptive?

A Well, congratulations on holding out till 23 – a major achievement these days!

Though the IUD (loop or coil, or whatever you like to call it) can be a wonderful method of contraception for some, it's important for women to realise that it may occasionally have disastrous side-effects. *And these side-effects are much more likely to happen in women who – like yourself – have never been pregnant.* One of the major risks in a 'never pregnant' woman is that of infection, possibly in part because many unmarried women have more than one lover.

If the infection gets to your tubes, it can make you sterile. So talk things over *very* carefully with your GP or family planning clinic before you elect to use an IUD.

Q I was fitted with some sort of IUD which was shaped like the figure '7'. Not long afterwards, I got a severe infection in my tube, and spent two weeks in hospital. Could the infection have been connected with the coil?

A Yes – though you might have trouble proving a 'cause-and-effect' relationship. But, as I've been saying in this column for years, pelvic infections are more common in women who use any type of IUD – including the now-famous Dalkon Shield.

Q My doctor said I could have an IUCD, but the clinic have offered me an IUD instead. What's the difference?

A There isn't any difference. People get a bit confused about this because of the fact that some doctors say 'IUD' (meaning 'intra-uterine device') while others say 'IUCD' (meaning 'intra-uterine *contraceptive* device').

There's no truth in the rumour that the letters 'IUD' stand for 'It's up dere!'

Make sure you understand about possible side-effects before you have an IUD (see previous question).

The IUD

'IUD' stands for 'intra-uterine device'. This description covers all of the many devices which are placed inside the womb, including the coil, the famous

IUD

Lippes loop, and the various copper devices.

Many millions of women world-wide rely on the IUD for protection against unwanted pregnancy. In the USA, however, its popularity has been limited by the sad occurrence of a number of disastrous infections in women who were using a brand called the Dalkon Shield.

That particular brand of IUD has long been taken off the market, but it must be admitted that there is a small danger of womb and tube infection with any type of IUD. Bear in mind that if the tube infection does occur and is left untreated, this could seriously affect your future fertility.

But the *common* side-effects of IUDs are:

heavy periods

prolonged periods

expulsion of the device.

Despite these and other much rarer side-effects, IUDs suit four out of every five women who try them. The insertion process takes only a few minutes; it's generally much easier and less uncomfortable if the woman has had children.

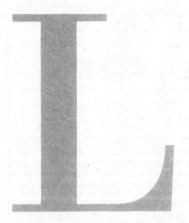

Lactation

Lactation really is the most amazing function. Despite the fact that breast-feeding temporarily became rather unpopular in the late 20th century, it's true that the vast majority of human beings who've ever lived have owed their survival to the fact that their mums lactated.

How does it all work? The interior of your breast is rather like a bunch of grapes. The milk is manufactured in those little sacs, and then it comes down a series of ducts into the reservoirs – between 15 and 20 little chambers which lie right behind your nipple.

During pregnancy, the sacs are stimulated by female hormones to grow and to get ready to produce milk. Some authorities reckon that this process makes the average woman add three pounds to the weight of her bosom during pregnancy. (Certainly, the late and much-missed Diana Dors used to say that becoming pregnant was the only way she knew for a woman to significantly increase the size of her bust.)

Small amounts of fluid may be secreted in late pregnancy, but it's not until you've been delivered of the afterbirth (placenta) that things really start happening. The placenta is a rich source of hormones, and the moment it's gone there's a remarkable 'all change' in the hormonal balance of your body.

In particular, the front part of your pituitary gland releases a hormone called prolactin to start stimulating those milk sacs to produce.

However, lactation probably *won't* go very well unless you're given the chance to put your baby to the breast, and let her/him suck firmly and frequently. It is suckling your baby which actually stimulates the pituitary gland (at the base of your brain) to produce both prolactin and — very importantly — oxytocin.

Oxytocin is another pituitary hormone. It works on the ducts so that the milk 'comes on down' — the rather startling sensation described by many women as 'my milk coming in'.

I can't really over-emphasise the fact that unless the breast is regularly suckled, your pituitary won't be stimulated — and therefore lactation will probably fail. That's why birth expert Sheila Kitzinger says that 'love play involving playing with the breasts and sucking and stimulating them is probably the best preparation for breast-feeding.'

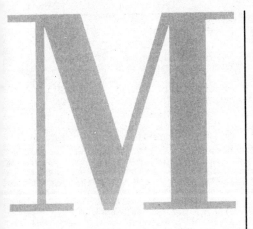

Q My wife is devastated by the fact that she has just had a breast removed.

She cannot believe that I still desire her. How can I convince her that this is so?

A Well sir, unfortunately many women do find it very hard to believe they are still loved and desired after losing a breast.

Ideally, ladies should have careful pre-operative emotional counselling before a mastectomy operation – but this doesn't seem to have happened in your wife's case.

So, I urge you to call on the services of that marvellous organisation, the Breast Care and Mastectomy Association; their counsellors and their literature may well help her. Write to them (enclosing sae) at: *26A Harrison Street, London WC1H 8JG.*

Meantime, all you can do is keep telling her that you love and want her very much.

The Menopause

Let's get the blokes out of the way first. *There is no such thing as a menopause in men.* After all, 'menopause' actually means 'cessation of the periods' – and I need hardly remind you that men don't actually *have* periods! The various symptoms which people are all too ready to attribute to a 'male menopause' are actually due to such causes as psychological stress and overwork – *not* to hormonal changes. For men, unlike women, are very fortunate in that the output of their sex hormones falls only very, very slowly over a period of 20 to 30 years from the 40s onwards.

Women, however, are different in that their sex hormone output falls very rapidly indeed at the time of the menopause (average age 49 in Britain). This can result in very trying symptoms.

All I need stress here is that the menopause does NOT mean the end of your sex life, or of your physical attractiveness or womanly beauty. You may not even get any 'menopausal' symptoms – like hot flushes – but if you do, these can usually be treated fairly successfully nowadays with hormone replacement therapy.

The menopause can be a blooming *awful* time for many women, but others sail through it without difficulty. A sympathetic and understanding husband and family can do much to alleviate the stresses and strains of the change of life. However, it's a PHYSICAL and not an 'emotional' one, so don't let anyone tell you different! Commonest symptoms are hot flushes, sweating attacks, and vaginal dryness.

Sex life, incidentally, should not be adversely affected by the menopause. In fact, many women find that once they are free of the nuisance of periods and (not long afterwards) free of the risk of unwanted pregnancy, life takes on the quality of a 'second honeymoon'.

How Should Periods Stop?

Most women are confused about this important point, and a lot of them think that heavy bleeding ('flooding'), or irregular bleeding is normal at this time. *This is a dangerous myth.*

There are only three ways in which the menopause should occur.
(1) periods stop suddenly and never return: or,

(2) they get less and less in volume until they cease altogether; or,

(3) they get farther and farther apart in time until they stop completely.

Bleeding between the periods or after intercourse, irregular bleeding, or very heavy bleeding are all abnormal. If you have these symptoms, consult your doctor, who'll probably do an internal examination. He may then send you to a gynaecologist for further tests.

Of course, the cause of the trouble may be something relatively minor, like fibroids or an erosion of the cervix, but only proper investigation will tell whether this is the case. The risk of cancer of the womb and of the cervix is so great at this age that it is essential for you to consult your doctor at the least suspicion of anything being wrong.

Bleeding *after* the menopause is also a potentially serious symptom – if it occurs, see your doctor as soon as you can.

Menopausal Problems

Menopausal problems affect hundreds of thousands of women – and can mess up their sex lives. However, the outlook for your love-life is generally good – mainly because this is in some ways the very sexiest time of your life. (It's widely reckoned that women reach the peak of their sexual performance when they're over 40.)

Common menopausal problems are:

hot flushes (referred to in the USA as 'hot flashes')

sweating attacks

dryness of the vagina.

All of these are due to a relatively sudden drop in hormone levels. *And all of them can be successfully treated by hormone replacement therapy (HRT) using female hormones.*

The hormones can be given by mouth or by implant under the skin. However, where the main problem is a dry, sore vagina which is making intercourse difficult, it's a widespread practice to give the woman a tube of vaginal hormone cream.

A few weeks of nightly application of this will usually restore her vagina to its previous healthy state – and love-making to normal.

81

There's a very slight danger that her partner will absorb some of the hormone through the skin of his penis. A few men have temporarily developed little breasts as a result of this unusual method of absorption, but the risk is pretty small (like the breasts).

Oral female hormone dosage should be very carefully controlled by your own family doctor, gynaecologist or menopause clinic. It is believed that, in the past, overuse of unbalanced hormone preparations (particularly in the USA) has led to cases of cancer of the lining of the womb.

But, quite obviously, management of menopause symptoms is *not* simply a question of replacing a few hormones. All women who have menopausal problems need love and understanding from their husbands, families and friends.

Note: If you're having trouble getting hormone replacement therapy (HRT) or regular check-ups, contact the Family Planning Information Service (01-636 7866), who will tell you the address of the nearest Menopause Clinic.

Menstruation

Nearly all women menstruate — as a rule, between the ages of about 12 and 49. A woman menstruates on average 13 times a year, so she has to put up with something like 480 periods during her lifetime.

A woman's first few periods are often painless. But once she has menstruated a few times, the odds are that she will get at least some pain. It's thought that at least five million women in Britain, and at least 25 million in America, suffer from some degree of period pain (or 'dysmenorrhoea', to give it its posh name).

It's also important to realise that at least a fifth of that number suffer from menstruation which is *too heavy* or *too prolonged*. This is why so many women (in contrast to men) become anaemic: they lose too much iron in heavy or prolonged periods, so that the blood becomes weak.

Happily, modern treatment *can* help a woman combat painful, heavy or prolonged periods. In particular, I have to say that the fact that there are countless millions of women on the Pill has made a great difference to the world-wide problem of period pain and appallingly heavy periods. Despite its possible side-effects, the Pill is remarkably good at:

abolishing period pain

lightening the menstrual flow

shortening the duration of menstruation.

But in view of the fact that menstruation causes women so many problems (you can't blame them for calling it 'the curse'!), you may ask why on earth a woman has to be bothered with it all. The reason is fairly straightforward. Each month, the womb builds up a rich lining, ready to receive a fertilised egg. This lining is filled with blood vessels. However, if *no* fertilised egg embeds itself in that rich lining (in other words, if the woman doesn't get pregnant that month), then her body's hormone balance 'tips' in such a way that the lining breaks up.

The break-up of the blood-rich lining naturally causes bleeding, and that's the period. The reason it looks a bit different from 'ordinary' blood is that it's mixed with debris and secretions from the womb lining.

Micturition

One function about which there's still considerable embarrassment is micturition. Even today, a lot of women (and indeed men) find it difficult to discuss the subject with their doctors – partly because they don't know any 'polite' term for having a pee.

Anyway, in an attempt to reduce the general embarrassment about this subject, let me explain just how micturition works. You have a urinary bladder which is located just in front of the upper part of your vagina. It's filled by two tubes (the ureters) which come down from your kidneys. And when it empties, the urine passes out through the short tube called the urethra.

At the outlet of the bladder, there are two tight constricting rings of muscle (called the sphincters) which prevent the urine from coming out till you want it to.

Normally, you are quite unaware of any sensation in your bladder until about 150ml of urine has accumulated in it (that's a little over a quarter of a pint).

At that stage, the nerves which run upwards from your

MICTURITION • MISCARRIAGE

bladder to your spinal cord and brain start sending a few mild signals – saying something like 'Listen, owner: we're going to have to do something about this in the next hour or two.'

But if more and more urine begins to accumulate in your bladder, you begin to feel discomfort. When the quantity reaches 600ml (which is a bit over a pint) the signals coming upwards become very urgent. If you tried to 'hold out' much longer you simply wouldn't be able to. Curiously enough, in pregnancy a woman *can* hold out much longer – the pregnant woman seems to have a sort of dispensation so that her bladder can hold at least twice as much.

When you finally decide that it's time to go to the loo, what happens is this.

One set of nerves relaxes the outer sphincter. Another set relaxes the inner sphincter – and makes your bladder contract. And that's it – you 'go'.

Finally, what *should* you say to your doc when you want to describe this important function? I would recommend either 'pass water' or 'pee'.

Q I have just suffered a miscarriage. Is there any way I could find out *why*?

A I'm so sorry to hear about this, as I'm sure it was distressing for you.

If it's any consolation, you're not alone: the recent *Delvin Report* suggested that almost one in five SHE readers have had 'a miss'.

In fact, about 20% of all pregnancies are thought to end in miscarriage. Usually the cause is totally unknown. So unless your doc has any suggestions, I think you may just have to write it off as upsetting but far from unusual.

Q This afternoon, my fiancé and I made love, and the condom split. After the tears and despairing laughter, we decided to go to my GP to ask for the 'morning after pill'.

My usual doctor wasn't free, so I had to see another one. To my indignation, she wouldn't give me the 'morning after pill' as it was against her religious beliefs about abortion!

Surely she has no right to mess about with my life in this way? Doctors aren't allowed to express their opinions like this, are they?

A I'm afraid that everybody is

84

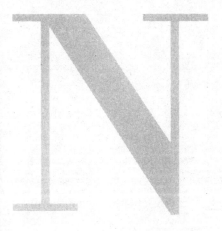

entitled to express their views — and that nobody can force a doctor to do something which is against their ethical or religious principles.

However, while I respect this doctor's views, it does strike me as quite extraordinary to equate giving a pill (about two hours after sex) with abortion.

Your letter indicates that you were planning to see your regular GP the following day, and I hope you did so and got the tablets.

Nowadays, all GPs have the facility to prescribe the 'morning after pill', and most are willing to do so. It's just a question of taking two tablets of something called Schering PC4 — and then two more in 12 hours' time.

Q I'm worried about the pink, circular area round my nipples.

This area is quite large, but when I'm cold and my nipples stick out, the pink disc shrivels up and looks really tiny.

I've never let any of my boyfriends see my breasts, because I feel so ashamed.

A No need for shame. The pigmented area round the nipple is *supposed* to shrivel up tightly when it's cold. So you're normal.

If you visit any of our chilly British nudist beaches this summer, you'll see that most of the women there have very small, retracted areolas. (And the chaps have their little problems with the cold, too . . .)

The Nipple

The nipple is one of the most sexually sensitive areas of the body – in both women *and* men. Some women can reach a climax through having just their nipples stimulated, though I don't know of any gents who can manage the same.

Anyway, let's get clear the basic anatomy of the nipple. Most people use the word wrongly: they think it means the *whole* of the pigmented disc in the middle of the breast. In fact, only the central bit which sticks out is called the nipple; the disc which surrounds it is called the areola.

The areola is quite sensitive too, but it doesn't have anywhere near as many nerve-endings as the actual nipple. The areola may be pink, brown or black –

depending on your general colouring. It can be anything up to five inches (12.5cm) across, and there's no 'normal' size. People are sometimes worried by the little blobs which often run round the areola, but these are perfectly normal structures called 'the tubercles of Montgomery' (no connection with the Field-Marshal, as far as I know).

The nipple itself contains the openings of the 15–20 milk ducts, plus the aforementioned nerve endings – which are directly connected to one of the most important emotional regions of your brain. That's one reason why suckling a baby *and* sexual stimulation of the nipple both tend to have an immediate emotional impact on a woman.

The nipple also contains a lot

Q Though I have large breasts, I have flat and underdeveloped nipples. Is there anything at all that I can do? I feel I am abnormal.

A Sorry to hear about this. The very latest results of *The Delvin Report* (our sex survey among 6,000 SHE readers) show that no less than 27% of respondents were unhappy about their breasts or nipples! However, *personally*, I reckon that if more women went to topless beaches and saw how other ladies are built 'up top', they'd be happier and realise that their bodies are *not* abnormal.

I do appreciate that you feel particularly badly about the flat-

of erectile tissue; in other words it can stand up, like a man's penis. Usually, both the nipple and the areola become much more prominent well before orgasm – but your areola loses its swelling very rapidly after a climax; the nipple usually takes quite a lot longer to go down.

Disorders

Inturning (inversion) of a nipple is common, and is *not* a disorder if you've had it all your adult life. If it makes breast-feeding difficult, then your midwife can prescribe you a 'nipple shell', which may help. But a sudden and unexplained inturning of the nipple *is* a potentially dangerous symptom, as it may indicate that a growth is pulling the nipple inwards. An urgent medical check is necessary.

Similarly, blood (or a brown discharge) coming from the nipple can be a danger sign. However, with luck it may only indicate a small papilloma (benign swelling) in a milk duct.

Finally (and I'm sorry to conclude on a gloomy note, but it is a very important one), a raw or weepy eczema-like patch on the nipple or areola in the over-45s must also be investigated *fast*, since it may indicate a malignant disorder called Paget's disease of the nipple. This has no connection with the more famous Paget's disease of bone, which is *not* malignant – Sir James Paget (1814–1899) confused everybody by being the first to describe at least four different diseases.

ness of your nipples. If you really want to have something done about them, then it would be possible to have them 'elevated' by a plastic surgeon – though I don't believe that you could ever get this done on the Health Service. Good luck.

Q I have 'inverted nipples' and would like to get them sorted out before I go topless sunbathing this summer. Is it possible to have them corrected by operation?

A Yes, ma'am. A good cosmetic surgeon could make your nipples stand out for about 500 quid or so per nipple.

But I would like to stress that it is a serious symptom if a nipple inexplicably becomes inverted during adult life – and it means that you must get yourself examined by a doctor fast.

Q I am a man, and I notice that I have slight soreness and pain on passing water – plus a hint of discharge.

I have had tests and do *not* have gonorrhoea. So what could this be?

Non-specific Urethritis

Also known as NSU or non-gonococcal urethritis (NGU), this is by far the most common sexually transmitted infection in males today.

In most cases, NSU appears to be caused by the relatively 'new' organism chlamydia. Some cases may be due to other bugs, notably one called mycoplasma. The symptoms in men are:

pain on passing water

discharge from the penis.

As we'll see in a moment, those symptoms are very like these of gonorrhoea, though NSU is generally regarded as a milder infection. It can, however, have very serious complications (e.g. arthritis) in a small number of cases. Also – and very importantly – it now seems very likely that NSU in a man can make his female partner ill, or even sterile, by giving her chlamydia. Unfortunately, symptoms in *women* tend to be vague or non-existent – though there may be fever and pelvic pain.

Fortunately, treatment of NSU with one of the tetracycline group of antibiotics is usually successful. You should refrain entirely from sex until cured.

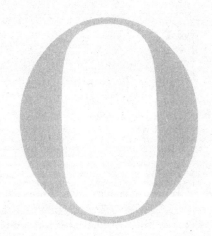It's important that everyone should realise that there's now a fantastically common sexually transmitted infection in this country – yet its name is not well known to the public.

It's called 'non-specific urethritis' ('NSU' for short – which must confuse certain German car manufacturers), and it's now actually more common than measles. It's usually caused by a bug called 'chlamydia'. Chlamydia isn't all that easy to test for, so many clinics simply treat men on the basis of the *symptoms* of NSU – discharge and pain passing water.

You have these symptoms, so you should now go to a VD clinic and get yourself treated immediately.

The Ovaries

Tucked away inside your pelvis, you have two ovaries. They're jolly little oval pinkish-white things, each about 3.5cm (1½") long and 2 cm (¾") across – just a bit smaller than a man's testicle, in fact.

The comparison with a man's "balls" is an apt one, because the ovaries are the exact female equivalent of the testicles, and are formed from the same tissue in the early human embryo. However, nature very sensibly tucks the ovaries away where they can't be damaged (would that she had done the same for us lads!).

Only someone with fairly long and fairly skilled fingers can feel them: they're just about palpable through the upper part of the side wall of the vagina – and some women do like having them gently stroked during love play.

Your ovaries probably contain about 100,000 eggs each, but only one egg is released each month, making a grand total of about 400 during your reproductive lifetime. Incredibly, all the rest go to waste!

Apart from releasing eggs (ovulating) the ovaries are also important sources of a woman's sex hormones – though not, curiously enough, the *only* sources. If the ovaries have to be removed, some female hormones are still manufactured in other parts of the body.

Ovulation

Ovulation means the release of an ovum (egg) from your ovary.

It happens once a month – usually about 14 days before the start of your period. A 'ripe' ovum bursts from the surface of your ovary, makes an extraordinary long jump across the enormous gap which separates the ovary from the Fallopian tube – and then belts down the tube on the off-chance of meeting an inquisitive little sperm coming up the other way!

Not too long ago, I was at a meeting which was being addressed by Robert Edwards, of Steptoe and Edwards fame.

He revealed that he has now found that ovulation nearly always takes place in the early afternoon.

Indeed, when his American patients come to Britain to

Disorders

Disorders of the ovaries are frequently difficult to diagnose, simply because of their inaccessibility.

CYSTS are very common, particularly in younger women. (Princess Anne had one removed a few years ago.) Many cysts produce no symptoms at all, but others can cause pain which can be mistaken for appendicitis.

By some weird quirk of nature, a few ovarian cysts when removed turn out to contain teeth (no kidding!).

Contrary to what many people believe, cysts of the ovary are not caused by the Pill. In fact, the Pill tends to protect you against them.

CANCER. Sadly, cancer of the ovary is quite common, and kills rather more women than the much better-known cancer of the cervix. The cause is not known, but again there is now evidence that the Pill helps to protect you against it.

Symptoms tend to be rather vague, and include persistent low abdominal pain, and bleeding after the menopause. Let me stress that the disease is rare under the age of 45.

Happily, there's a very new screening test for cancer of the ovary – it's done by ultrasound, is painless and takes only ten minutes. Unfortunately, the few ovary-screening units that offer the test are fairly swamped with patients at the moment.

undergo the 'test-tube baby' technique, he finds that they're ovulating at about 3pm *New York time*. But after a month or so in Britain, they start ovulating at around 3pm Greenwich Mean Time.

Edwards' announcement prompted a rash of speculation that early afternoon might be the best time to get pregnant. But don't make any arrangements for post-lunch love-making yet –

for if you think about it, the ovum usually takes a day or two to make that journey down the Fallopian tube. So provided you make love *around* the day of ovulation, there's a good chance of conceiving.

Now let's just look at what causes ovulation.

Your ovaries are about the size of small walnuts, and each of them contains the incredible figure of about 200,000 potential eggs. As a rule, only one of them ripens each month (if *more* than one ripens, you may get twins).

The release of the egg is caused by a hormone signal which travels each month from your pituitary gland (at the base of your brain) to your ovaries.

Emotional stresses – or even a sudden change of work or diet – can interfere with that hormone signal, which explains why irregularity of the menstrual cycle often happens in women who've had some sort of recent upset.

You may possibly have noticed that you get a slight pain in the lower tum midway between periods; this is actually caused at the moment of ovulation by the egg being released. It's called *mittelschmertz* – which is simply German for 'middle pain'. For some women, it's a useful sign that they really are ovulating.

Women: Failure to Ovulate

For a variety of reasons, an awful lot of women do not ovulate (produce an ovum). This can be the case even though they may be having periods. So one of the first things to do in most cases of failure to conceive is to try to check whether the woman

is ovulating.

A simple and cheap way of doing this is for her to take her temperature every morning over a spell of several months. If she is ovulating, her chart should register a 'kick'.

Admittedly, temperature charts can be difficult for even the most experienced doctors to interpret. In some cases, it's necessary to check whether ovulation is occurring (and – most important – *when*) by one of these methods:

hormone tests

ultrasound scan of the ovary

biopsy (sampling) of the womb lining

laparoscopy (inspecting the ovary with a telescope-like device pushed through a small cut in the abdomen).

Obviously, these methods are much more expensive (and, in most parts of the world, more difficult to obtain) than the simple temperature chart procedure.

Once a woman knows that she's ovulating – and *when* – then obviously she should make love around that day in order to conceive. But if the tests show that she's *not* ovulating, then these days there's still hope for

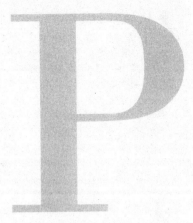

her.

Failure to ovulate can very often be successfully treated with the famous 'fertility drugs' – which stimulate the ovary to produce eggs. Most of these drugs mimic the action of the natural hormones which are produced by a woman's pituitary gland, which should make her ovary produce an ovum each month.

Unfortunately, as you probably know from the newspapers, use of certain fertility drugs does often over-stimulate the ovaries, so that they produce *too many* eggs. The result is a multiple pregnancy; indeed in a few cases, the fertility drugs have had the startling effect of giving the woman up to eight babies.

I'm afraid that the survival rate of the babies in these extreme cases of multiple pregnancy is low.

Obviously, infertility specialists try to control the dose of fertility drug very carefully so that if possible only one, two or at most three babies are produced at a single pregnancy.

Usually (though not invariably), a woman who has been desperately trying for a baby over a period of many years is usually only too delighted if she ends up with twins or even triplets!

Q I am in my mid-50s, and last year had a pelvic floor repair operation. Prior to the operation, the surgeon did warn me that intercourse might be difficult.

It's not difficult — it's *impossible*, because I am now so tight! Will things improve with time, or would you advise me to get my husband one of those inflatable dolls?

A Well, congratulations on your sense of humour, ma'am! A well-performed pelvic repair op usually makes intercourse better — not worse; you should go back to the surgeon, or get a second opinion. A 're-fashioning' operation might be necessary. But it's possible you could be helped by either female hormone cream or vaginal relaxation exercises — or possibly through the use of graduated dilators which stretch the tissues. Good luck.

Q I am an 18-year-old male and I am worried because my penis is bent to one side when it is erect. I could not see my doctor about this.

A Well, I'm afraid you're going

The Pelvic Floor Muscles

Lots of people don't really understand what the pelvic floor muscles are. Indeed, recently I had a slightly surreal conversation with an otherwise highly-informed woman who thought that pelvic floor exercises were so called because you had to do them on the floor!

The pelvic floor is a cleverly interwoven basket of muscle which forms a network that supports the organs in the pelvis — including the womb, ovaries and bladder. You can get a rough idea of the size and shape of the muscles of the pelvic floor simply by holding your two hands palms upwards in front of you. Then slide the two hands together, so that the fingers interlock. The resulting shallow basin is quite like the pelvic floor. Imagine that it's supporting your pelvic organs and that there are two apertures in the basin, through which pass the vagina and the rectum.

It's very important for all women to know about this pelvic floor musculature because in so many ladies, childbirth leads to serious *weakening* of these muscles — with unfortunate consequences for love-life and health. Repeated childbirth and *difficult* and *prolonged* labours are particularly likely to do this. As far as her sex life is concerned, a woman is likely to find that her vagina seems to have become slack and loose.

Furthermore, severe weakness of these muscles can lead to *prolapse* (descent of the womb); much more frequently, it simply causes problems with urination and the woman may find that she has embarrassing incontinence, especially when she coughs or laughs.

Gross weakness of the pelvic floor muscles can usually be put right, with one of a variety of surgical repair operations. Obviously, it's much better to avoid surgery altogether, and this can be done by means of pelvic floor exercises.

Every woman should do these exercises daily for several months after the birth of a child. Any woman who feels that her vagina is a little too loose can do these exercises – they are quite good fun, and they may prevent the need for a vaginal repair operation later on in life. The exercises develop the muscles just where they surround the vagina, and where they grip the penis during intercourse.

Indeed, the exercises can and should be done during intercourse: this is enjoyable, and your partner will find it pleasant too. Once these muscles are strengthened, you'll discover that doing the exercises creates an agreeable sort of 'milking' sensation in his male organ. But it's no good just doing the exercises during love-making. As with any other 'muscle building' exercises, *you need to do them for about 20 minutes twice a day – over at least six months.*

You can do the two exercises while you're at work, or pushing a pram, or sitting in the bath – no one will know you're doing them. Here they are:

Exercise one: make a real effort to tighten up the *front* part of your pelvic muscles, by 'tightening up' as if you were trying to stop yourself passing water. Hold the contraction for 10 seconds, then release for 10 seconds. Continue for 10 minutes.

Exercise two: make a similar effort to contract the back part of your pelvic floor muscles by 'tightening up' as if to hold back a bowel movement. Again, maintain the contraction for 10 seconds, then relax for 10 seconds – repeat for 10 minutes.

The Penis

Now to the organ which so many people get concerned about: the penis.

It's surprising that this particular organ generates such a lot of emotion, embarrassment and even outrage. For after all, it's a somewhat unimpressive little structure, comparing rather unfavourably in dimensions with a decent-sized *andouillette*.

However, one has to face the fact that many men and women do have hang-ups about the penis. In the case of men, vast numbers have an extraordinary obsession about penis size – and are firmly convinced that their own is too small. In the case of women, a surprising number of females feel frightened or disgusted by the idea of a close encounter with a male organ.

You may be surprised to hear it, but some wives are so emotional about this matter that they cannot bring themselves to touch their husbands' penises.

Perhaps life would be easier if everybody understood a few of the basic facts about this organ. The penis is the male equivalent of a woman's clitoris. It's equipped with a great many 'pleasure receptors' which, when stimulated, produce very agreeable sensations in the man's brain.

The average penis in its non-erect state is quite a bit smaller than most people imagine. In general, it measures between 8.5cm (just over 3ins) and 10.5cm (just over 4ins) – but it varies a lot, depending on the weather.

Masters and Johnson have discovered a curious fact of which few men are aware. Though penises vary quite a bit in size in the non-erect state, they are

to have to – because no one else is going to straighten this out for you.

In fact, your doc will probably send you to a specialist called a urologist, who will be able to tell you whether there is anything wrong, or whether this is just a slight variation from normal.

Urologists see a lot of blokes who are worried because their penises develop a bend when they become erect. Since a specialist can hardly examine a man during an erection, some urologists actually ask men to bring in a Polaroid photo of the erect penis – so that they can assess the degree of bend.

Please don't worry too much about this – but you definitely do need a medical opinion.

nearly all about the same size when they are erect. So though many males feel inadequate about the size of their penis, this is all quite unnecessary — especially as most women are not remotely interested.

The penis is a very simple structure in comparison with the female genital organs. It consists of three 'cylinders' of tissue, which are capable of filling with blood (thus causing an erection).

On the end of these three cylinders is the cone-shaped glans, which is the most sexually sensitive part.

The only other thing to say about the penis is that contrary to what so many women (and men) imagine, it's actually a pretty clean structure. Provided a man washes regularly under his foreskin (if uncircumcised) there should be nothing 'dirty' about it.

Q What's the best treatment for period pain?

A It's usual to start with aspirin or paracetamol, or one of the vast number of formulations based on them.

But, if that doesn't work, some

Period Problems

The menses, or periods, begin at about the age of 12 on average, though many girls experience the first menstruation as early as 10 or as late as 16. (If the periods start before 10, or if they haven't started by the 17th birthday, always check with the doctor.) Menstruation continues until the change of life, which means that the average woman will have something like 400 periods.

One still finds patients who think that the female cycle is somehow linked to the calendar (or even to the Moon!), and who therefore expect their periods to arrive on the same day of every calendar month. In fact, the menstrual cycle is usually considerably less than a full month in length — 26 days from start to start being about the average. Quite a lot of women have cycles as short as 16 days, or as long as 40 days, and some have periods only once every few months or so.

Irregular and Heavy Periods

It really doesn't matter all that much how long the menstrual cycle is. (There is nothing especially 'right' about a 26-day or

97

PERIOD PAINS

28-day cycle, as a lot of people think.) All that is important is that the periods should be reasonably regular, and that blood loss should not be excessive.

If the periods are irregular, you should always consult a doctor. Nobody need expect their period to come with split-second timing each cycle, but a woman ought to be able to forecast the arrival of her menses to within about two or three days.

Bleeding between the periods or bleeding after intercourse are possible *danger signs* and must not be ignored. See your doctor, who will probably perform an examination and, if necessary, refer you to a gynaecologist.

Heavy periods are not only a nuisance but are liable to cause excessive loss of iron, with resultant anaemia. It is largely because women have periods that they're so much more liable to anaemia than men are.

It's hard to say what constitutes heavy loss in any individual case, but if you are getting 'flooding' (*i.e.* if tampons and towels don't seem to be coping with the flow very well), or if regular bleeding goes on for more than six days each month, or if you are getting unusually pale or unusually tired and breathless, then it's definitely

doctors believe in prescribing an anti-spasmodic called Buscopan. A successful trend in recent years has been to try anti-rheumatic drugs such as Ponstan and Naprosyn.

However, by far the most successful abolisher of period pain in Britain is the Pill. Most younger women who suffer from dysmen find that a correctly chosen brand of the Pill wipes it out.

Some people are not very keen on taking the Pill, and ask for other hormones instead. But the truth is that these are usually Pill-type hormones under another name – and probably have similar side-effects.

Commonsense measures include a hot water bottle on the tummy or the back – and gentle massage of the same areas.

A feminist group recently raised a few eyebrows by suggesting that rubbing one's own clitoris would help. Acupuncture is also useful, but rather less fun.

Q How I wish I could just bring on my period each month on exactly the day when *I* want it!

It would be nice just to 'flush

best to check with your doctor. He will examine you, and probably do a simple blood test to find out if your body's iron stores have been depleted by excessive menstrual bleeding. If so, it shouldn't be too difficult to put things right. The Pill and similar hormone preparations can, of course, have side-effects — but they are very, very effective in treating heavy, prolonged and irregular periods.

Painful Periods

Pain with periods can be very troublesome indeed. In the past, it was something of a fashion for (male!) doctors to say that much of the distress was purely psychological, and that if the girl would only pull herself together all would be well. This was (literally) bloody silly.

Period pain is often absent when the menses first start, but may begin a few months later. The reason for this is that in the early menstrual cycles, there is often no ovulation (see below), and in many patients ovulation seems to be necessary for menstrual pain to occur.

This is why taking the Pill is often a cure for painful periods, since it suppresses ovulation. That provides an effective

everything away' every four weeks, and not have to worry endlessly about contraception.

Why haven't you doctors come up with anything convenient like that?

A Sorry! In fact, there is a French tablet which will do more or less what you say. It's called RU468.

It does give women the power to control their own fertility — and to bring on a period when they want one. But, unfortunately, as with every other drug, there are side-effects. *And because the tablet is regarded by many people as an abortifacient, there's bound to be a heck of an ethical row about releasing it in Britain.*

Pro-life MPs have recently started asking questions about the new drug — and they appear to have obtained assurances from the manufacturers that RU468 WON'T be sold over the counter to British women. It also seems likely that a British woman who wants to use it will have to get two doctors to sign an Abortion Act form first.

If this is true, my personal forecast is that feminists will try to smuggle it in from France.

method of treatment, but in younger girls with only relatively mild period symptoms, it's often best to begin treatment with simple analgesic drugs. A large number of preparations are now available for the relief of period pain, and the doctor will often try quite a variety before he finds a suitable one. If pain is bad, there should be no hesitation about taking the day off school or work and retiring to bed. A hot water bottle clasped to the tummy will often provide a lot of relief. Anti-inflammatory drugs like Ponstan may be helpful.

Ovulation and Periods

You need to understand the relationship of ovulation (the release of an egg from the ovary) to the menses, since ovulation is the time at which conception occurs.

Most of the time, in most women, ovulation happens a little before the half-way point of the menstrual cycle. For a woman whose periods are 26 days apart, therefore, the likeliest time for conception is about 11 to 13 days after the start of a period.

Ovulation varies a lot, however, and there is no way of being *sure*. A slight backache is sometimes a clue to the fact that it is taking place. Some patients take their temperature every morning before getting up and record the results on a chart. A little 'kick' upwards on the graph (preceded by a slight dip) very often occurs on the day of ovulation.

It is also possible to buy 'conception-day indicators', simple calculating devices into which one feeds data concerning the length of recent menstrual cycles. As a way of reckoning the conception day they are not as effective as the temperature chart method.

The time at which conception is *least* likely is just before and during the menses. Some people call this time the 'safe period', but this is a bit misleading; there are hundreds of thousands of children in the world who owe their existence to the fact that their parents believed in the 'safe period'! All that can be said is that it is probably safer than any other time of the cycle. Many Catholic women (and others) swear by the 'Billings' version of the 'safe period', in which you plot the nature of your vaginal secretions on a daily chart.

Q Is it true that the Pill gives you cancer of the liver? I have been on it for three years, and have always been very careful to have regular check-ups. My doctor assured me that I was on a 'low-dose' brand which could not possibly cause side-effects.

But last week I read a newspaper report which said that doctors had found that it caused liver cancer.

I made an appointment to see my doctor and asked him if I should have tests for liver cancer, but he just laughed at me.

A Oh, dear – a rather unfortunate response, I fear. But, in fact, nobody who is taking the Pill needs to have tests for liver cancer.

However, papers in the *British Medical Journal* have suggested a possible (but very, very minute) risk of liver cancer from long-term use of the Pill. Naturally, this has caused some newspaper headlines.

Though this complication is very rare, any woman who gets persistent tummy pain or jaundice while on the Pill should see her doc urgently.

However, one final point: despite what your doc says, there's no such thing as a Pill which 'could not possibly cause side-effects.'

Q I get very depressed on the Pill. Have you any suggestions?

A Well, if you definitely feel that the depression is due to the Pill, then either come off it or switch to a totally different brand.

Alternatively, some women who become depressed on the Pill do feel they can combat it by taking pyridoxine (vitamin B_6). Your doctor may be willing to prescribe this, or else you can buy it without prescription at the chemist's.

But although there's a lot to be said in favour of the Pill, it's crazy to keep on taking it if you get depression or other severe side-effects.

Q My girlfriend has decided that she shouldn't go on the Pill. Would it be safe if we made love unprotected within ten days of her period starting?

A No – if you do this, she will in all probability get pregnant. If you want to use the 'rhythm method', then go and get some medical advice about how to use it properly. (And I warn you – it isn't easy.)

The Pill

The Pill remains fantastically popular in most western countries. For instance, in Britain there was a time quite recently when a startling *one in three* of all women of child-bearing age was taking it!

But although the Pill has been in widespread use for many years (it was invented in 1956), there are still worries about it – and new facts are constantly coming to light about it. So it's better not to go on it unless you've fully discussed any doubts you may have with your doctor or clinic.

Having said that, I have to add that the Pill is probably the most outstandingly successful contraceptive of all time. Taken properly – which means for 21 days out of every 28 – it will give you virtually 100% protection against pregnancy.

It does this because it contains two female-type hormones (an oestrogen and a progestogen). These affect the pituitary gland – at the base of the brain – so that it no longer sends out signals telling your ovaries to ovulate.

Side-effects

Most women who go on the Pill get no side-effects. But during the first few packs a substantial number do experience headache, nausea, breast tenderness, weight gain or bleeding between periods.

Serious side-effects are rare. But cases of thrombosis (clots) can be *fatal*. The danger of this happening is much greater in smokers, in more mature (35-plus) women, and in those with certain other risk factors. *Heavy smokers should never take the Pill*. Even moderate smokers should try to give up this dangerous habit.

The relation of the Pill to cancer is very complex. At the time of writing, it *appears* (and I stress the word *appears*) that the Pill probably helps protect you against two types of cancer – of the ovary and the womb lining – but *may* increase the risk of other types, including cancer of the cervix and (in younger women) of the breast.

Make sure you discuss any worrying reports with your doctor or clinic – and take advantage of regular smear tests for cancer of the cervix which all Pill-prescribing doctors or clinics can arrange.

Finally, after all these warnings, do bear in mind that the Pill does have certain very *good* effects. In particular, a well-chosen brand should make your periods painless, shorter and lighter.

The mini-Pill

The mini-Pill is used mainly by women who no longer wish to take the Pill (e.g. the over-35s) and by breast-feeding mothers (this is because, unlike the ordinary Pill, it doesn't suppress milk production).

It is not a low-dose version of the ordinary Pill, but is a quite different thing, containing only one hormone (a progestogen) instead of two.

At the moment, it does appear to be much 'milder' than the ordinary Pill, and complaints of side-effects are much lower. Disruption of the periods is the chief possible side-effect: they may become too far apart, or irritatingly frequent!

The mini-Pill seems to work *mainly* by thickening the secretions in the cervix, making it difficult for sperm to get through. You must – repeat *must* – take it *every single day at about the same time, without any breaks at all.*

It's at maximum effectiveness about 6 to 8 hours after you take it. So if you usually make love in the late evening, you'll get the best protection by taking your mini-Pill each day at around 4 pm.

One word of warning: although the mini-Pill's reputation is as a very mild contraceptive, it *is* nonetheless a hormone. This means that its long-term effects will not be known for a long time to come. If in doubt, discuss any anxieties you may have with your doctor or clinic.

The Vaginal Pill

In the mid-1980s, world-wide interest was aroused by the announcement that a Brazilian researcher, Professor Coutinho, was giving the Pill by the vaginal route. (It can easily be absorbed by the vaginal tissues.)

This may seem a bit strange, but the basic idea is, in theory, not a bad one. Taking the Pill in this way does prevent one of itscommon side-effects, namely nausea.

I had the entertaining experience of being at the meeting where Professor Coutinho first presented his findings at the Royal College of Obstetricians and Gynaecologists in London, at which he suggested that a major British trial of his vaginal Pill should now take place.

A questioner from the floor leapt up and declared that this method of adminstering the Pill would *not* be acceptable to British women. She added that if anyone set up a trial in the UK, there would be a high rate of drop-out.

'*Drop-out?*' thundered Professor Coutinho, misunderstanding completely. 'Certainly not – my Pills do not drop out!'

The New French Monthly Pill

In 1985, the world was startled by reports from France of a new once-a-month pill, which a woman could simply use every 28 days to 'clear out' he womb. It was alleged to be 100% effective. Quite understandably, this idea aroused a lot of indignation among people who regarded the new French invention as a licence to carry out do-it-yourself abortion – which would make it unacceptable to a very large number of women. Indeed, in late 1988 'pro-life' pressure forced the manufacturers to stop making it. Then the French Government ordered them to carry on!

I have talked to Professor Baulieu, the French inventor of this new pill – which at the moment is usually known as RU468. He recently told me that while he has high hopes for his invention, it's probably only about 95% effective at the moment, and it has to be used in combination with strong drugs called prostaglandins.

This makes do-it-yourself administration rather more difficult. Also, both RU468 and the prostaglandins are powerful drugs; all past experience suggests to me that there could be long-term side-effects.

Q I want to go on the Pill, and would like to know what is the safest, please.

A Unfortunately, it's still impossible to say which of the 25 or so brands of the Pill is the safest.

It is known that the old 'high-dose' brands of Pill were more dangerous from the point of view of causing thrombosis. But after I complained about them in this column some years ago, a question was asked in the House of Commons. Soon afterwards, they were all taken off the market.

Today, most Pills are 'low dose', though a few are 'medium dose' (50 microgrammes).

Most GPs and Family Planning Clinics tend to prescribe the low-dose pills for the majority of women.

Q I am on the Pill and I'm going abroad soon. Will I be able to get the same Pill in other countries?

A Probably not, but there are equivalent brands. For details of brand names, contact the International Planned Parenthood Federation on 01-486 0741.

Q I keep forgetting to take my Pill. What should I do in order to avoid getting pregnant?

A If you keep forgetting to take it, then maybe you should be on some other form of contraception. But obviously, everyone forgets their Pill occasionally.

The latest FPA advice on how to cope with this common situation is as follows:

If you're more than 12 hours late taking your Pill, you could be at risk of pregnancy. You should take *extra* precautions (like using a condom – or not having sex) for the next seven days.

If you missed the Pill during *the last week* of your packet, then it's best not to have a break between that pack and the next one.

Q Is it really true that the Pill can be taken vaginally?

A Yes, it is true – and taking it by this rather bizarre route does mean that you avoid one of the very common side-effects of the Pill – namely nausea.

But the danger is that you wouldn't be able to get the Pill far enough up; there's also a risk that its coating might not dissolve quickly enough for the contraceptive to be effective.

And your chap might be unfortunate enough to absorb a dose of it when he made love to you! So please, I warn you, don't attempt to try this lark without medical supervision.

THE PILL

Q I will soon be 35, and therefore unable to take the Pill any longer. I don't want to use one of those coil things, and my husband dislikes any kind of rubbery contraception. Can you suggest anything?

A Well, vast numbers of women are encountering this problem at the moment – now that doctors are tending to take many women off the Pill at about 35. But the No Pill After 35 rule certainly isn't an absolute one. The risk of being killed by the Pill doesn't suddenly shoot upwards on your 35th birthday; in reality, it seems to increase very slightly throughout your 30s and 40s. So some women do stay on the Pill for a little while after they're 35. But when the time comes to *stop* taking the Pill, the solution for many women these days is the mini-Pill. This is not – repeat *not* – a low-dose version of the ordinary Pill; it's a quite different thing. Basically, it's a tablet that contains just one hormone, instead of the two hormones in the ordinary Pill. It's free of oestrogen – a fact which appears to make it less risky. Indeed, at the time of writing (touch wood) no one has ever had a fatal thrombosis caused by the mini-Pill. So talk to your doctor or clinic about the possibility of switching to the mini-Pill.

Because so many people are muddled about just which brands are mini-Pills and which *aren't*, I'm going to list the available ones here. They are: Femulen; Micronor; Microval; Neogest; Norgeston; and Noriday.

Q Whenever I go and see my doctor to get a prescription for the Pill, she seems to be obsessed with how much I smoke. Is there some connection between smoking and the Pill?

A Yes – I'm constantly amazed at how few people realise this. Smoking is not only dangerous in itself, but it also increases the risks of the Pill considerably. One major British study suggests that if a Pill-taker starts smoking, she may become eight times as likely to die of a heart attack or stroke.

So if you want to go on taking the Pill, the best thing is to give up the dreaded weed altogether. Smoking is a mind-bogglingly stupid habit – and especially so for somebody on the Pill.

Q A year ago I was forced to stop taking the Pill because my blood pressure had risen considerably. Since then, my boyfriend and I *have not* enjoyed having to use the diaphragm.

Is there any type of Pill which is freer of side-effects?

A Well, it'd certainly be worth asking your doctor to tell you about the 'mini-Pill'.

That's the one-hormone only Pill which you have to take every single day, but which is generally milder than the ordinary Pill.

I can't guarantee that it'd suit you, but it's worth considering.

Q I am thinking of going on the Pill, since most of my girl friends seem to be on it. But does it cause cancer?

A At the time of writing, there isn't as much worry about the relationship between the Pill and cancer as there was during the last 'Pill scare'. Also, it has become clear that the Pill almost certainly protects women to some extent against two particular types of cancer.

But the Pill certainly hasn't got a clean bill of health, and I have to admit that there are still serious question marks over the link with breast and cervix cancer.

This is a bit worrying, since three million British women still take the Pill and are theoretically at risk (it remains the most popular method in the UK, in fact).

So if you do choose the Pill, you should take even more care than other women to do two things: (a) check your breasts regularly for lumps; (b) have regular smears done.

But remember, this should be your own decision. Clearly you shouldn't go on the Pill just because your friends are on it.

Q Is it true that as I am a contact lens wearer, I must not take the Pill?

A Nope. This is a common myth, but there's no reason why contact-lens wearers shouldn't take the Pill.

However, some contact users do find difficulties with their lenses when they first start the Pill. This is probably because of increased fluid retention in the eyeball, but it's not usually much of a problem.

Q I'm going on the Pill. How often should I have check-ups?

A Opinions differ, but most

authorities say that you should be seen by a doc or nurse every six months — particularly to discuss 'risk factors' like smoking and high blood pressure.

Frequency of internal examinations and breast checks depends a lot on what facilities are available in your area. At many hard-pressed NHS clinics 'internals' tend to be done about every three years. Breast checks may be omitted altogether, I'm afraid, so it's best to make sure that you know how to do your own check-up each month.

Q I have recently picked up what appear to be white worms round my bottom. They make me itch at night, and are very uncomfortable. I am too embarrassed to go to my doctor, so could you please tell me what to do to get rid of them?

A These are almost certainly threadworms (pinworms), which are very common. If you have any children, you may have picked up the worms from them.

They live in the lower part of the bowel, and come out of the bottom at night to lay their eggs on the skin — which is why the itching is always nocturnal.

There's been recent discussion in medical journals about how the threadworms KNOW that it's night-time? (After all, it's always dark up your bottom.)

Anyway, what happens next is that you scratch your underneath parts — and get eggs trapped under your fingernails.

If you're not careful, it's then easy to transfer the eggs to someone else's mouth (eg: on food) — or to re-infect yourself via your own mouth.

I think you should see your doc to get the diagnosis confirmed — especially as the odds are that the whole family will need treating (usually with a drug called piperazine).

Q I have very bad PMT which is driving my husband up the wall. My doctor has been treating me for several years with Cyclogest suppositoires. Is there anything else?

A Yup. Cyclogest *suppositoires* are OK, but they're not everybody's cup of tea, so to speak.

Other treatments for PMT include the hormone dydrogesterone, Vitamin B_6, diuretics ('water pills'), and Efamol capsules. I suggest you talk these possibilities over with your doc.

There's also an advisory service for people with pre-menstrual tension, which stresses the alleged nutritional basis of the problem. They have produced a book 'Beat PMT Through Diet' – £5.99 Ebury Press, but I don't know of any very convincing evidence that it will help you.

Q I went to my doctor recently for a post-natal check, and was surprised that he did not examine me internally.

A That's very odd indeed. I take it that he wasn't one of these SAS-type doctors – trained to get in and out without anyone noticing.

More seriously, you do need an internal examination after you've had a baby, just to check that everything's back to normal. (You may also be due for a smear.)

If it's awkward to return to this doc and demand an internal, then

Pregnancy and Sex

It's quite common for women suddenly to lose interest in sex either during pregnancy or immediately after it.

This reaction may be partly due to hormone changes. It can also be linked to the stress and tiredness which affect so many women during pregnancy, child-birth, and the months afterwards.

There may also be a psychological element. A number of women do have a feeling deep down that sex is all right for young women – but that once you become a mother (or a mother-to-be) then you really shouldn't enjoy it any more!

In many cases, this loss of interest cures itself – especially if the couple talk about it together and the man adopts a sensible and sympathetic attitude.

Incidentally, the great weight of medical opinion nowadays is that there is no reason at all why you shouldn't make love during pregnancy. Provided there are no abnormalities in the course of the pregnancy (e.g. bleeding) there seems to be no harm in making love as late as you like. A recent study in the *New England Journal of Medicine* seems to indicate that babies of couples who made love late in pregnancy are just as healthy as those of couples who didn't.

However, when you get very big, sex in the orthodox positions can be uncomfortable. You may prefer to restrict yourselves to love-play when pregnancy is far advanced.

I suggest you make an appointment with your local Well-Woman or Family Planning Clinic (I've checked, and there's one not far from you). If you explain the situation, they'll most likely be pleased to oblige.

Q I am horrified to find that my doctor has just diagnosed a prolapse. Is it due to having too much sex?

A A prolapse is a general sort of collapsing downwards of your internal sex organs, caused by weakness of the supporting tissues.

It's *not* caused by sex – but by childbirth (and particularly *repeated* childbirth).

It is slightly less common than it used to be, mainly because women are having smaller families these days. Exercises may help in mild cases – such as the excellent ones provided by the self-help groups which have recently sprung up in women's gym classes.

But if your case is more severe, I'm afraid you'll need a 'tightening up' operation, to take in a few 'tucks' and try to restore you to your former state of beauty.

Q I read your recent article about the prostate gland. I am a man who has had this operation, and I would like to say that what no one ever tells you is that after it has been done, the ejaculatory function is lost. The feeling at

Prostate Gland

This is a gland about the size of a large chestnut which lies at the neck of the male bladder. There is no exactly corresponding structure in women, though recent research suggests that the G-spot in women is a very similar organ. The prostate gland produces a liquid that forms part of the seminal fluid.

The urinary passage goes right through the prostate, and the unfortunate consequence of this is that enlargement of the gland will block the flow of urine from the bladder, either completely or partially.

The cause of the enlargement of the prostate is not known, but, like greying of the hair, and stiffness of the joints, it's probably just another consequence of ageing. It doesn't seem to affect sexual function.

The patient with an enlarged prostate usually notices that he has some difficulty in producing a good stream of urine, and that

orgasm is still there, but there is no ejaculation.

A Well, you're quite right, sir. If the prostate gland is removed (or if a substantial amount is 'nibbled away' with a surgical instrument)

you do not ejaculate. This is disappointing and irritating to quite a few men.

It's a pity that the surgeon didn't explain this to you beforehand – though I think that most men would have gone ahead with the op anyway.

sometimes it may be very difficult to 'get started', particularly when the bladder is full. Most patients are obliged to get up once or twice at night to pass water.

There is also a risk of *acute retention* developing; in this condition, no urine can get out of the bladder at all and prompt treatment is necessary.

Treatment of an Enlarged Prostate

GENERAL. Many mild cases of prostatic enlargement can be kept in check by simple means. If you have a moderately enlarged prostate, you should avoid drinking large quantities of fluid, particularly alcohol, tea and coffee, all of which tend to increase the flow of urine. (These drinks are quite all right in moderation, however.)

Make sure you empty your bladder regularly – say, every one to two hours, and especially

before setting off on long journeys. The worst possible thing to do, for instance, would be to have several pints of beer before a long, unbroken car ride home on a cold night – this would be inviting an attack of acute retention.

Another important point to remember is that prostate sufferers are particularly liable to inflammation of the bladder or cystitis and, in fact, any kind of urinary infection. So, if you get pain and discomfort on passing water, see your doctor as soon as possible, so that he can send a carefully collected specimen of urine to the lab for culture.

SURGICAL. When prostate trouble gets too bad, surgery is essential. About one prostate patient in four eventually needs an operation. It's now often possible to carry out what's called a TUR (or transurethral resection), which simply involves pushing a slim telescope with a cutting device up the urinary passage, and nibbling away bits of the prostate so as to make the passage wider. But the surgeon may operate to remove the *whole* prostate gland.

This procedure (prostatectomy, as it's called) at one time used to be very dangerous, and very distressing for the patient. Nowadays, it's a straightforward and safe business, though the few days after the operation are not usually much fun.

Most patients do very well, however, and are out of hospital within about two weeks. A month

or so of convalescence will be required. Urinary control should usually be regained shortly after the operation.

With luck there will be only partial interference with sexual function, and some men, because of improved general good health, actually enjoy happier marital relations after the operation. Seminal fluid will no longer be produced at orgasm, which means that the man will probably be unable to have further children. Since most patients are at least in their late fifties, and have long completed their fami-

Pruritus

Pruritus literally means itching, but the word is often used to mean itching of either the vaginal opening (*pruritus vulvae*) or of the back passage (*pruritus ani*).

Vulval and Vaginal Pruritus

Itching of the vulva and vagina is a trying and embarrassing symptom for many women. There are various possible causes. It may be necessary to examine the urine for sugar (which might indicate diabetes). Bacteriological swabs from the vagina should usually be sent to the lab,

particularly if there is a discharge present, as is often the case. Frequently, examination of these swabs will reveal the presence of thrush (also known as Monilia or Candida) or of another organism called *Trichomonas vaginalis*, sometimes confusingly known as TV.

Other causes of irritation in this area include fungus infections, and other skin inflammations, as well as allergy to vaginal deodorants, contraceptive foams, soaps and bubble baths.

Anal Pruritus

Irritation of the back passage is

lies, this is not usually of any consequence.

Cancer of the Prostate

When a patient who has symptoms of prostate trouble seeks medical advice, the doctor should always do a rectal examination, since this enables him to feel the size, shape and texture of the gland with his finger. If the gland feels craggy and hard, cancer may be present, but I must stress that cancer is *rare* compared with ordinary benign enlargement of the gland.

Cure of prostatic cancer can be achieved by complete removal of the gland. Some patients are treated with hormones.

Some doctors, especially in the US, feel that all males over the age of 50 should have a yearly rectal examination to detect both benign and malignant disease of the prostate, as well as disorders of the rectum itself. Lives could probably be saved by this sort of universal screening, but the costs would be huge.

a very widespread problem, especially in men. A lot of doctors think that psychological factors play a part in at least some cases, but they could be wrong! Physical factors include inflamed piles and anal eczema, which is very common and responds well to steroid ointments.

Threadworms and fungus infections can produce intense pruritus, and the symptoms can also follow the taking of antibiotics by mouth. Over-vigorous wiping of the anal region after defaecation can also lead to irritation, as can sitting for far too long in hot baths.

Q My lack of hair in the pubic area has made my life a misery.

Why? Because my second-ever lover spread the word around our town that I was hairless in this region, and it made me a 'local joke'.

Since then, I have never been able to go out with anyone, and I have become very lonely and depressed.

A I'm so sorry to hear about this. It's appalling that your former lover treated you like this.

If you really have practically no hair around the 'pubes', then you may be suffering from a hormone

113

deficiency, which might be put right.

I can't guarantee this – but I do think that you should ask your doc if she'll refer you to an endocrinologist (that's a gland specialist) to see if hormone therapy would help.

If not – well, bear in mind that many men actually LIKE a girl to have 'bare pubes' and enthusiastically beg their partners to shave it all off! So have courage – I'm sure all will be well.

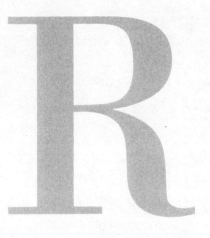

Q Would it be all right to shampoo my pubic hair? I always feel that mine is rather thick and 'crinkly', and that this will put men off.

A I'm sure it won't – after all, pubic hair is supposed to be deep and crisp and even (as they say).

But there's no reason at all why you shouldn't shampoo your 'pubes' with ordinary hair shampoo – and put conditioner on as well if you like!

In fact, I'm surprised that some enterprising shampoo manufacturer hasn't already come up with a special brand for this area.

Stop Press: As this book went to press, I learned that pubic shampoos have just reached the shops.

Q Is it true that there's a new, 100% reliable version of the 'rhythm method?'

A Nope. But large companies have made significant advances towards developing a 'home test', which would enable a woman to pinpoint her own ovulation day.

I reckon it'll be at least several years before they get the bugs ironed out. But when they do, it'll be a great boost for the 'rhythm method' – not to mention the Catholic Church.

Rhythm – and Other 'Natural' Methods

'Natural' methods are the only ones which are at the moment acceptable to the Catholic Church. It's true that in recent years there has also been more interest in them among non-Catholic couples – partly as a result of understandable worries about the Pill and other hormonal contraceptives.

However, the proportion of couples outside Catholic countries who use natural methods is still very low indeed – probably less than 1%. To be frank, I am not surprised, because the failure rate of these methods is very high, except among those who are extremely well motivated.

Natural methods fall into two groups: rhythm, and lactation.

Rhythm Methods

Rhythm or the 'safe period' techniques depend on avoiding love-making at the time when the woman is most likely to be fertile. This tends to be in the 'middle' of the menstrual month – in other words, roughly halfway between periods.

Unfortunately, however, women *can* ovulate at almost any time of the month, so if you want to use the rhythm method, it is best to employ some method that will help you to identify the 'danger days' with reasonable accuracy.

Quite soon now, science will find a cheap and convenient way in which any woman can pinpoint her day of ovulation. But until then the best ways of estimating your safe and 'danger' periods are:

the temperature chart method

the Billings method.

The *temperature chart method* relies on taking your temperature every morning, and plotting it

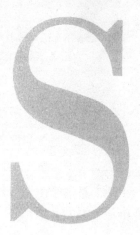

with great accuracy on a specially designed chart.

The *Billings method* was invented by two Australian doctors, John and Evelyn Billings, and involves plotting the nature of your vaginal secretions on a chart. The idea is that, on certain days of the cycle, when the vaginal secretion is clear, slippery and 'stretchy', fertilization is very likely, and sex should therefore be avoided.

Learning to identify the nature of your secretions correctly takes time, patience, intelligence and commitment. It also requires careful *training* by someone who knows what they're doing. So do not attempt the Billings technique by yourselves. If you decide to try it, both of you should attend one of the special 'Billings Clinics', which (in the UK) are often run in co-operation with Catholic Marriage Advisory Councils.

Salpingitis

This is inflammation of the Fallopian tubes, which run from the ovaries to the womb. It is caused by infection with germs, and may be either acute or chronic (*i.e.* long-lasting).

Acute Salpingitis

This is a common cause of acute abdominal pain. The chief symptoms are pain in the lower abdomen (either right-sided or left-sided, depending on which tube is involved) and fever, with a temperature of perhaps 102°F (38.9°C). There will often have been a vaginal discharge and some menstrual irregularity in the preceding few weeks.

The patient is usually admitted to hospital. With the correct antibiotic treatment, the outlook is good and most people are well on the road to recovery within a couple of weeks.
See also: CHLAMYDIA.

Chronic Salpingitis

This is a long-standing inflammation, which may follow infection of the tubes during childbirth or abortion (miscarriage). It may sometimes be due to gonorrhoea, especially where the original infection produced no symptoms. Another common cause is Chlamydia.

The features of this condition are variable but include intermittent pain low in the abdomen, vaginal discharge, irregular and painful periods, and sterility.

The skilled care of a gynaecologist is essential. Surgery is sometimes helpful, but prolonged medical treatment may be required.

The Shot

In the west, a very small number of women use the Shot (also known as the 'Jab'), though it has been employed on a wide scale in Third World countries. It has long been fully legalized in Britain, though in America the FDA have reiterated their objections to it over many years, because of doubts about possible long-term side-effects.

It's an injection that prevents you from getting pregnant, and gives virtually 100% protection. The injection is a hormone of the progestogen type (that is, like one of the two hormones in the Pill). By far the most common brand worldwide is Depo-Provera (also known as med-roxyprogesterone acetate). A less widely used brand is Noris-terat (norethisterone oenanthate).

Women's groups in many countries have got very indignant about Depo-Provera, and have waged highly successful cam-paigns against its use. I must say that I have to agree with two of their objections.

Firstly, the drug has all too often been given to women 'routinely' without any mention of possible side-effects. (Many women in Britain were at one time given it post-natally without ever realizing that it was Depo-Provera.)

Secondly, there does seem to have been a small but disturbing

A Low Sperm Count

Unfortunately, vast numbers of men do have a low sperm count (or no sperm at all) even though they're perfectly capable, virile lovers.

That's why the simple, inexpen-sive test of doing a sperm count should be carried out very, very early in the investigation of a couple with infertility problems (and certainly long before the woman is subjected to any uncomfortable, expensive or time-consuming tests).

All the man has to do is to provide a sample of his seminal fluid in a hospital specimen jar. He should climax directly into the container and not, as many men do, in a condom – because the rubber may harm the sperm.

The specimen jar should be taken within an hour or two to the hospital laboratory, where it will be examined under a micro-scope and a count made of the number of sperm in it. Repeat tests are often necessary, mainly to exclude technical errors.

Why is the sperm count so often found to be low? The sad answer is that in most cases we simply don't know.

Sometimes a man's sperm out-put is low (or even zero) because of past infection of the testicles – particularly by mumps. Some-times it's low because of injury to the testicles, or because of a recent spell of ill-health. Also, certain drugs can depress sperm production, as can some hor-

tendency for a few white doctors to regard it as an acceptable way of controlling black fertility for so-called 'sociological' reasons. In one notorious case in Britain, a doctor gave a black woman the Shot while she was under a general anaesthetic (and therefore somewhat unlikely to give her consent); his rather unusual justification for this was that he had done it in the interests of the taxpayers.

On the other hand, I have to say that the Shot is a very effective contraceptive, which is actively *demanded* by a small number of women for whom no other method is suitable. Its chief known side-effect is menstrual chaos. Any woman who opts to use the Shot must understand that her periods may become very frequent, or disappear.

mone disorders. However, very often the cause remains a mystery.

Treatment

If the sperm count is repeatedly *nil*, then I am afraid that there is usually little that can be done. The couple should consider AID (Donor Insemination) or adoption.

However, if the sperm count is merely on the low side, then there *is* hope. You'll get detailed advice from your infertility clinic, but possible ways of improving the sperm count include:

wearing loose, cotton underwear instead of tight, synthetic-material briefs (the latter increase the temperature of the testicles, and this depresses sperm production)

having surgical treatment for any *varicose veins* which may be present just above the testicle (a common condition)

having hormone treatment to stimulate the testicle – though this method is of very limited success

'saving up' love-making – in other words, abstaining from sex for a week or so before the woman's ovulation day, in order to build up the sperm count.

Q I have one child, but after trying for three years for another one, we found that my husband's sperm count is low. The hospital advised him to dip his testicles into cold water before intercourse. This is rather chilly on the bottom! Is there anything else we can do to increase his sperm count?

A Well, for a start I'm afraid that there's no point in carrying out this somewhat masochistic ritual *immediately* before love-making, as sperms take about six weeks to mature inside the male body. So, as far as anybody knows, the 'cold water treatment' will only improve your man's sperm count in about 42 days' time. But wearing cool, unrestricting underpants certainly is important.

Another useful measure was revealed in a recent paper in *The Lancet*. Three Australian doctors say that if you get a man really excited, and give him plenty of love-play before intercourse, then he'll produce more sperms. They got this idea from the world of agriculture, where, they state, it's well known that 'preliminary teasing of a bull results in samples of better quality'!

The Sponge

The Today Sponge (sold in some countries under the name 'Prelude Sponge' or 'Collatex Sponge') came onto the market in various countries, including the UK and the USA, in the mid-1980s. It's a vaginal sponge, and the interesting thing about it is that it is very acceptable aesthetically to many women who appreciate its non-messy qualities.

It's a soft disc of sponge, about 5 cm (2 in) across. The sponge comes already impregnated with spermicide, so you don't have to add any when you want to make love.

All you do, in fact, is to take the Today Sponge out of its pack, moisten it, and then gently tuck it into the topmost part of your vagina – using the tips of your index and middle fingers to ensure it fits tightly against the cervix. Neither you nor your partner should be able to feel it during intercourse.

The sponge has to be left in place for at least six hours after intercourse, though it can be left in for up to two days if necessary. When the time comes to remove it, you simply hook your finger round a polyester tape which is attached to the underside.

The Today Sponge is disposable, and you can buy it over the counter in a chemist's shop (without a doctor's prescription).

But how safe is the Today Sponge? There have been claims that it is 98% effective. But anyone who has studied the history of contraception knows that claims like that nearly always need to be taken with a generous pinch of salt.

Ms Walli Bounds of London's Margaret Pyke Centre, who is probably the UK's leading expert on intra-vaginal contraceptives, is sceptical of the figures which have been put forward. She warns that the true failure rate of the Today Sponge may well turn out to be higher than that of any of the reliable methods which are widely used at the moment, such as the cap.

In the USA, a New York congressman has claimed that the Today device may cause cancer. But the US National Institute of Health flatly denies these allegations, and the FDA itself has given its approval for the device to go on sale.

There have also been suggestions that the sponge could cause the dangerous Toxic Shock Syndrome (the overwhelming infection which is usually associated with tampon use). But so far I know of no cases in Britain.

Sterility

About 10 to 15% of marriages have trouble with fertility. Inability to have children is a very distressing problem for any couple. Of course, not everyone can expect to have children exactly whenever they want them, but if you've been trying for, say, 12 months without success, then it's as well to seek help.

The family doctor will usually refer patients to a gynaecologist who specializes in the treatment of infertility; many hospitals run (badly overcrowded) infertility clinics these days. Alternatively, simple tests are often done at Family Planning Clinics.

At these clinics, the first problem is sometimes found to be that the wife is still a virgin and the couple are not really having intercourse at all! This may sound astonishing, but even in these supposedly well-informed days there are a surprising number of husbands and wives who simply don't know how to set about having a child (though they usually think that whatever they are doing is how babies are made).

Assuming that this problem does not apply, however, the next thing is to decide whether the couple are trying at the right time of the month – *i.e.* ovulation, which is usually about 14 days before the start of a period. If you have intercourse each day for three or four days running at about the time of ovulation, then the chances of pregnancy are much better.

If this fails, full investigation of both parties is necessary. Even today, men tend to blame infertility on women, but the fact is that in many marriages it's the husband who is sterile, even though he may be potent or indeed highly virile.

The gynaecologist will therefore arrange a lab test on the husband's seminal fluid, mainly to see how many sperms it contains, and if the individual sperms are active and normally formed.

A post-coital test is also useful. The woman is examined shortly after intercourse, and a check is made as to whether the husband's sperms are surviving in the secretions of the vagina and cervix.

The woman also needs full investigation, of course. She may have to have a D and C (dilatation and curettage), or scrape of the womb lining. Very often, the specialist will test whether her Fallopian tubes (which carry the eggs, or ova, from the ovaries to the womb) are blocked or not. This is checked by a simple procedure in which a little carbon dioxide gas is blown through the tubes from a narrow catheter inserted into the vagina. X-rays of the tubes can be carried out by injecting a radio-opaque dye in the same way.

Both these procedures are more comfortable under general anaesthesia, but they can also be performed without an anaesthetic. And the technique of laparoscopy (in which a slim telescope-like device is used to

Sterilisation

In most western countries (and many developing ones) the use of sterilisation, both female and male, has increased dramatically in recent years. A very large number of couples are choosing sterilisation once they have completed their families.

As for female sterilisation, the first thing to understand is what it does. The point of the operation is to block the woman's Fallopian tubes in some way, so that the sperm cannot get to the ovum.

This can be done by cutting

inspect the internal organs) can be of great help in investigating infertility. An ultrasound 'scan' of the lady's ovaries may also be helpful.

Treatment

If some disorder of the female genital tract is present, it can often be treated satisfactorily, and pregnancy may follow within a few months. If the Fallopian tubes are blocked, however, there may be a considerable problem, though some surgeons are beginning to achieve encouraging results with Fallopian-tube surgery.

And of course, the British pioneers and others all over the world have engineered the births of thousands of 'test-tube babies' – babies who are conceived in a laboratory dish from the husband's sperm and the wife's 'egg' or ovum. The fertilised

ovum is then put into the womb *from below* – thereby by-passing the diseased or missing tube. The newer 'G.I.F.T.' technique involves placing sperms and an ovum in the wife's Fallopian tube.

In many cases of female infertility, particularly those linked with hormone imbalance, the new 'fertility drugs' may be very helpful.

When infertility is due to the husband, the outlook is not usually very hopeful, though there are ways of raising low sperm counts. If there is no prospect of his fathering a child, he and his wife should consider whether they want to have a baby by AID (artificial insemination by donor). An increasing number of gynaecologists are willing to arrange this procedure, and couples who have chosen it are usually very happy with their baby.

through the tubes and tying them off, or by clipping them with a device like a very firm plastic paperclip. The effectiveness of sterilisation is very *nearly* 100%, but, as with any operation, occasional failures do occur.

The two common methods of

carrying out the procedure are:

traditional sterilisation

laparoscopic sterilisation.

'Traditional' sterilisation requires a longer stay in hospital. It's done through an incision – perhaps 10 or 13 cm (4 or 5 ins) long – in the lower part of the abdomen, round about the top of the bikini line.

Laparoscopic sterilisation is the newer and much more minor operation. It's done with the aid of the slim, telescope-like viewing device called the laparoscope. This is pushed through a very tiny incision near the navel, while a 'tube-clipping' instrument is pushed through another very small incision in the woman's side.

Quite obviously, most women would prefer to have this newer operation, but it's not available everywhere in the world; not all women are suitable for it; and there is a slightly higher failure rate (i.e. pregnancy rate) than with traditional sterilisation.

Q I'm thinking of getting sterilised. Is it true it can have masculinising effects?

A Nope. Sterilisation is a simple piece of 'plumbing work' on your tubes. So it shouldn't have any hormonal effects, or put hair on your chest. There have been suggestions that it can make the periods a bit heavier, but so far there's no proof of this.

Syphilis

The most serious of the venereal diseases – apart, of course, from AIDS. Fortunately, it's rare nowadays in Britain, and other types of VD (for instance, gonorrhoea and NSU) are much more frequently encountered. Promiscuous homosexuals are at risk, however.

Syphilis is caused by a germ called *Treponema pallidum*. It can always be cured, if it's caught in the early stages. If it's not properly treated, however, the long-term consequences (which include insanity and death) are quite horrifying. Fortunately such late complications rarely occur these days, partly because most people go to a 'Special Clinic' as soon as the symptoms appear. A few patients are still unwise enough to think that the disease will go away by itself – but it won't.

Symptoms

Syphilis is acquired by having sex (though not necessarily actual intercourse) with an infected person. (*N.B.* In many countries, though not in all, there is a very high risk of infection in having sex with prostitutes.) Very occasionally, a person with a syphilis sore on the lip may infect others simply by kissing.

The first symptom occurs nine to 90 days after exposure. A firm, painless sore develops on the genitals (or sometimes on other parts of the body, *e.g.* the lip or nipple). In women, there is a danger that the sore may sometimes be too far inside to be noticed.

The sore is usually smaller than your fingernail. A small amount of discharge may come from it. The nearby groin glands will probably swell up. After a variable period of time, the sore will go away. This does not mean the disease is cured – it isn't.

In the secondary stage of syphilis, which is usually a few weeks later, there may be a spell of general ill health, with sore throat, skin rashes, mouth ulcers and fever.

The tertiary (late) stage of syphilis occurs years later. Its appalling effects on the brain, heart and other organs need not be described here. These complications will *not* occur if you have sought treatment in the early stages of the disease.

Treatment and Prevention

Patients are sometimes tempted to treat themselves with 'borrowed' drugs because they are embarrassed about going to the doctor, but this is foolish – treatment is a specialised business. If it is to be adequate, proper lab tests have to be carried out.

In order to obtain these tests, you really need to attend the confidential Genito-Urinary Medicine Clinic (that's the new name for 'Special Clinic') at your nearest large hospital. You will probably be given a course of treatment lasting approximately two weeks, and it's vital that you don't abandon it part of the way through. You'll also be asked to return for further tests at a later date, and you'll be given printed cards to hand or send to anyone you have slept with.

Anyone who has syphilis (or any other form of VD) should on no account have sex with anybody until they are cured.

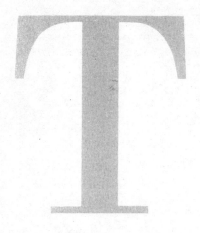

Q I'm going on a nudist holiday with my daughter this summer and we both want to know what ladies do about 'sanpro'.

Little strings or pads ruin poolside elegance. How do naturists cope?

A Quite easily, ma'am. Menstruating naturist women wear bikini bottoms or shorts.

The fact is not generally known,

The Testicles

It's fairly important for a woman to have a working knowledge of the male testicle — if only because it's so awfully easy for her to hurt it in bed! So be careful where you put your knees . . .

The testicle (also known as the testis) is an incredibly pain-sensitive part of the male body. This fact is vital to remember if you're *attacked* by a man. If at all possible, hit him as hard as you can in the testicles — and then run, because the disability is only temporary!

The testicle is, of course, the source of the millions of tiny sperm whose aim in life is to unite with a ripe ovum from the woman's ovary and so form a baby. Sperm, which are pro-

simply because 'nudist' magazines prefer, for some reason, to print pictures of people who are totally naked. Also, some naturist ladies tuck the little blue string just inside.

Q I lost a testicle when I was young, but am now happily married, with a good sex life and two children.

However, I feel that I am living with a deformity, and I would very much like to 'stand up and be counted' with other men! So, could I have an operation to put in a 'dummy' testicle?

A Yes, though you wouldn't get it on the NHS. The cost would be considerable, and there'd be an additional charge for the plastic prosthesis, which feels and looks very much like a real 'ball'.

As with any operation (especially

duced by the testicle, find their way up through a man's 'plumbing' in order to be ejaculated at the moment of climax. Anything up to 500 million of these are produced in a single orgasm.

But what actually happens to the testicles as a man gets sexually excited? Well, they're drawn upwards so that they press hard against his body. The work of Johnson and Masters indicates that if his testes do *not* do this, then he probably won't reach orgasm.

The two testicles have another function, which is to produce the male sex hormones, which give the secondary male sex characteristics of hairiness, muscularity, aggression, and so on.

Each testicle is rather like a flattened ping-pong ball in shape and size. Average dimensions are about (4 cm) (1¾ ins) long, 3 cm (1¼ ins) deep, and 2½ cm (1 in) thick.

Testicles occasionally have to be removed because of accident or disease. These days it's possible to replace a lost testis with a plastic one, which feels very like the real thing.

Although testicles are pain-sensitive, men do like them to be held by women – but gently! You shouldn't actually rub your partner's testicles; but if you hold them gently – particularly during intercourse – you'll find he'll appreciate it.

a rather unusual one) you should weigh up the risks of something going wrong before you finally choose to go ahead.

Q I have appalling thrush, and all my doctor treats it with is an interminable course of Nystatin, which is messy and stains my pants orange. Isn't there any other treatment?

A Yup, there is, ma'am. Nystatin is actually a good, reliable remedy, but you have to use it for 14 days — and, as you rightly say, it does have the unfortunate 'side-effect' of staining your knickers an unpleasant colour.

Here are some other drugs which are available and which can be used just as a single dose of one vaginal tablet: Canesten 1;

Test-tube Babies

The test-tube baby technique is one of the most brilliant medical advances of recent years. It has now enabled well over 1,000 childless women to have the babies they so much wanted.

Invented by two determined and clever men, British researchers Dr Robert Edwards and the late Patrick Steptoe, the technique is basically an ingenious way of getting round the all-too-common problem of blocked tubes.

It's important to realize that it isn't usually of help with other causes of infertility, as people often think.

The Steptoe technique is really a method of bypassing the blocked tube. The surgeon removes a ripe ovum from the woman's ovary, using a

telescope-like device known as the laparoscope.

Then the ovum is incubated in a glass dish, along with sperm provided by the husband. One of the sperm fertilises the ovum — and not long after the fertilised ovum is inserted into the woman's womb, via a slim tube passed up through her vagina.

Remember, however, that at present the technique is very expensive. Furthermore, at the moment only a minority of attempts succeed. If you're paying for each attempt, you could ruin yourself financially.

Still, it's undoubtedly a great step forward in combating infertility. (By the way, the 'test-tube baby technique' is something of a misnomer, since at no stage is a test tube involved in any way.)

Thrush

This is by far the most common vaginal infection in most countries. It's a fungus which causes:

intense soreness of the vagina

itching

an annoying discharge, which is usually creamy white.

In men, thrush usually produces no symptoms, but some men become red and sore. However, the sex partner of a woman with thrush is very possibly *carrying* it. Both partners should use an anti-fungal cream, and she should also use anti-fungal pessaries (vaginal tablets).

If thrush keeps recurring, your urine should be checked for diabetes. Thrush is more common in diabetics, and some diabetic males have to be cir-cumcised if it keeps giving them trouble.

If you think you have thrush, you should go to a doctor and have a vaginal swab taken, to confirm the diagnosis. The doctor will usually give you both anti-fungus cream for your exterior surfaces, and anti-fungus pessaries (vaginal tablets) to clear things up inside.

If you've read what I said above about hygiene, you'll appreciate that you should also avoid: tights, nylon pants, hot baths, *men* – at least until the condition is cured!

In recurrent cases, Pill-users may have to consider switching to another contraceptive.

Note: if you develop thrush, this does *not* mean that your partner – or indeed you – have been unfaithful.

Ecostatin-1; Gyno-Daktarin 1; Gyno-Pevaryl 1.

Also, you can now take oral tablets for severe thrush: these include Nizoral and the newly released Diflucan.

And don't forget the practical anti-thrush measures: avoid hot baths; don't wear knickers; avoid promiscuous blokes; make your man use an anti-thrush cream – or else give him a liberal local application of yogurt!

Q You recently said in SHE that yogurt could be used as a last resort in treating thrush. But is it harmful to get it into the vagina? And is it safer to stick to natural yogurt, rather than the fruit-flavoured kind?

A It's quite safe to put yogurt into your vagina as a treatment for thrush, though it's quite tricky to do. But I don't think you should use the fruit-flavoured kinds, because they tend to have all sorts of odd particles in them.

Indeed, about ten years ago I remember being summoned by an agitated family planning nurse to view a patient who had 'red specks all over her cervix, doctor!' Of course, the lady had been filling herself up with raspberry yogurt – and the 'specks' were the pips.

Q I suffer from a 'tipped womb' which I believe a lot of other women have too. Is it true that there's some special position in which it would be easier for me to conceive a baby?

A Yup. Women with 'tipped' (that is, retroverted) wombs are as common as left-handed ones. It just means that the womb points in a backwards direction instead of forwards.

If you're retroverted and having trouble in conceiving, then it's a proven fact (albeit a little-known one) that the best position to use when making love is kneeling on the bed with your bottom stuck up in the air.

I suppose that's what you'd call a hot tip. Good luck!

Q You have in the past stated that *Trichomonas vaginalis* can be transferred to women by men. But how on earth does the *man* get treated?

A Well, *Trichomonas vaginalis* (TV) is the second commonest cause of vaginal discharge, after thrush. It does go back and forth between women and men, in ping-pong fashion. So the male should *always* be treated as well, even though he won't usually have any symptoms.

Regrettably, often the husband/boyfriend doesn't get treated – with the result that the woman keeps on getting the discharge back again.

So any woman who is diagnosed as having TV should ask the doctor for Flagyl (or similar) tablets to give to her partner – and make him take them! Doctors may be unwilling to prescribe Flagyl if male partners are not on their list – so in that case, blokes must go to their own doc.

130

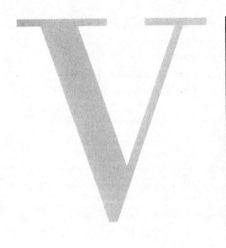
Vagina

The vagina, or 'front passage' as it's often quaintly called, is the wide, spacious, moist and well-cushioned channel which leads from the exterior up to the neck of the womb.

The word 'vagina' is Latin for 'sheath', and the reason for the name is of course the fact that the vagina provides an ideal 'sheath' for the penis.

There are many disorders of the vagina, and some of them can be extremely distressing for a woman. In this particular sphere, far too many patients suffer in silence. If you have some sort of vaginal trouble, the golden rule is to go and see your doctor before things get any worse. Don't delay because of embarrassment. The doctor will examine you and, if necessary, order lab tests or send you to see a gynaecologist. Family Planning Clinics provide another source of advice, as do Well Woman clinics.

Vaginal bleeding

Any type of vaginal bleeding other than the blood loss associated with completely regular periods needs assessment by a doctor.

BLEEDING DURING PERIODS (MENSTRUATION). Heavy

menstrual blood loss ('flooding') and irregular menstruation can readily cause anaemia, and should be treated as soon as possible.

BLEEDING BETWEEN PERIODS. Intermenstrual bleeding or bleeding after intercourse (even if it's only 'spotting' on the underclothes) may be a serious symptom. A full gynaecological examination is advisable. See your doctor within two or three days. But 'spotting' can also be due to an inappropriate brand of Pill (and is normal during the first couple of months on the Pill).

BLEEDING AFTER THE MENO-PAUSE. This too may be a serious symptom and needs immediate gynaecological assessment. Again, consult your doctor at the earliest possible date.

BLEEDING IN PREGNANCY. In early pregnancy (up to five months), bleeding is usually due to a threatened or actual miscar-riage. In late pregnancy, bleed-ing may be due to various causes, but must always be reported to your doc.

Vaginal and Pelvic Infections

These are so common that the great majority of young (and not so young) women these days get them at some time or other. These infections do seem to have become much more frequent since the advent of the permis-sive society.

That's hardly surprising, because it seems likely that all of them can be spread by sex – at least some of the time. Other factors which have made vaginal infections so much more common in the last 30 years are:

wearing tights (some organisms – especially thrush – *love* the warm conditions under a pair of tights)

wearing nylon underwear (same effect)

the fashion for frequent hot baths and Jacuzzis (which also prom-ote hot, moist conditions)

the widespread use of the Pill (which seems to make you more liable to thrush)

the widespread use of antibiotics (which also promote thrush)

Fortunately, most vaginal infections aren't serious – though they can be an irritating nuisance and badly mess up your sex life!

However, *deeper* pelvic infec-tions – which attack the tubes – can be very serious, and can even make you infertile. This is in fact a common cause of infertility today.

Vaginal Irritation and Discharge

IRRITATION. Vaginal irritation usually occurs together with discharge (but see also PRURITUS). DISCHARGE. One of the commonest of all symptoms, and one that causes a great deal of worry – often unnecessary worry.

It's important to stress that, from puberty onwards, a certain amount of vaginal secretion is completely normal. A lot of teenage girls don't realise this. Because they're often embarrassed about consulting their own doctors, they deluge newspaper and magazine advice columns with letters about this problem!

The vaginal fluid should be thin and reasonably clear; it has a natural aroma, the presence of which does not indicate a need for the use of douches or vaginal deodorants. The rate of secretion of the fluid varies from time to time and increases markedly when sexually aroused.

So when does a discharge need medical attention? Basically if it's thick, if it's yellow, green, brown or red, if it's irritant or associated with soreness or pain, or if it smells offensive.

Causes of discharge include disorders of the cervix (neck of the womb), and particularly cervicitis, cervical erosion and cervical polyps. Other common causes are infection by thrush and by the trichomonas parasite.

It's worth knowing that lately we've discovered that certain 'new germs' can cause vaginal discharge. A very common one is called *Gardnerella vaginalis*, which causes a greyish discharge with an embarrassing smell. It's treatable with Flagyl tablets. Also, never forget that a forgotten tampon can be a cause of vaginal discharge.

If you have one of the types of discharge outlined above, see your doctor. He should examine you and may send swabs to the lab for examination. If necessary, he should arrange an appointment with a gynaecologist.

Most types of vaginal discharge and irritation respond promptly to adequate treatment, though recurrences may occur in some cases. In view of the recent emergence of 'new' vaginal infections (like Herpes), if in doubt don't hesitate to go to a 'Special' or 'Genito-Urinary', clinic.

VAGINA

Q I am a teenage virgin. For some years I have had vaginal discharge, but my doctor doesn't seem to know what to do about it. Is there anywhere else I could go?

A Yes – there's a branch of the Brook Advisory Service for young people in your city: have a look in the phone book. But if you're a virgin, it's unlikely that there is any very serious cause for this symptom. (Most cases of serious infection are, I'm afraid, caused by sex.)

Q For over a year now, I've suffered with an extremely smelly vaginal discharge. Every swab and smear my doctor has taken has been negative, so I am at my wits' end.

A Sorry to hear about this. My best suggestion is as follows:

Quite often, an offensive discharge is caused by anaerobes, common germs which may not show up on conventional tests. It's characteristic of these organisms that they produce a distinct smell, which is offensive to the woman and (less frequently) noticeable to her partner.

Fortunately, anaerobes can be done in by oral tablets called Flagyl. An alternative is to use Flagyl *pessaries*, to be inserted into the vagina every other day.

Offensive discharge caused by anaerobes is common, and the fact that Flagyl cures it is not all that well known. In fact, recently I heard of a case in which a woman who'd had a very trying, offensive discharge for many years was only cured when by pure chance her dentist prescribed Flagyl for an anaerobic infection of her gums.

Q I have a fishy smelling discharge of the type which you mentioned in SHE earlier this year.

I was delighted when I read your article, because you said it could be treated with a tablet called Flagyl. (My GP had been unsuccessfully trying to treat it with antibiotics.) When I told him about the article, he gave me Flagyl, which cured the discharge.

But now it's come back again. Is this connected with the fact that I've been unfaithful to my husband? I'm afraid I dare not tell my GP this.

A Well, yes; you may well have been re-infected, either by your husband or by your lover.

I want to stress that Flagyl (also known as metronidazole) is *not* a cure-all for every type of vaginal

134

discharge. Nor will it take away the slightly fishy smell, which – for many women – is both healthy and normal.

I don't know what your doc actually diagnosed. But if you really feel that you can't go back and tell him the truth about your sex life, then I reckon you should go instead for a confidential chat and check up at a Genito-Urinary clinic.

Q For a long time, I've been extremely bothered by adverts for vaginal products which contain local anaesthetic.

I have always been led to understand that use of a local anaesthetic in this area could result in becoming sensitive to such things. Isn't that so?

A Yes, I'm afraid you're right. Local anaesthetic is used in some commercial preparations – with the specific idea of 'numbing' vaginal irritation or soreness.

Expert gynaecological opinion is against the use of these products – because (fairly obviously) if you've got something wrong with your vagina, you need to get it treated, not anaesthetised!

Also, you're quite right in saying that the application of a local anaesthetic can occasionally result in extremely painful sensitivity reactions.

Q I have recently been treated with Flagyl for a vaginal infection, presumably trichomonas.

But my husband has simply refused to take the same tablets, because he says 'he would know if *he* had any infection'. Would he?

A How remarkably silly of him. As I keep saying in SHE, women who have this common vaginal infection are all too liable to get it back again *if their sexual partners don't take the pills too.*

Tell your husband that men who carry trichomonas *don't* have symptoms. I think you'd be very unwise to have sex with him till he's agreed to take the tablets.

Q I hope to go water-skiing this summer. But is it really true that there are some special dangers for women?

A I fear so. There have been a number of cases in which the jet of water coming up from the ski has penetrated the woman's vagina, and caused serious injuries.

Nor is it just the women who're at risk: there's been at least one case of a chap who got a nasty squirt up his bottom and had to spend some time in hospital recovering.

However, I'm told that there is virtually *no* danger if you wear a proper protective wet-suit, with the usual strap underneath. But under no circumstances should anyone go water-skiing in a bikini – or (as I believe sometimes occurs among the jet set) in the nude. This is asking for what us doctors call 'trouble down below'.

Q After four children, my vagina is terribly loose, so that love-making is not as satisfying as it should be. I can't face the thought of a repair operation (which you mentioned recently in SHE), so what can I do?

A I must have had hundreds of letters recently about laxness of the vagina. (I hasten to add that when I speak of vaginal laxity, I mean the muscular, rather than the moral variety.)

Here are two useful tips for readers who find that their vaginas have become a little slack: (1) Try making love with your thighs *together*; this helps you to grip your man much more firmly; (2) If your bloke is fairly adventurous, get him to experiment with gently putting a finger inside you *at the same time*

as he's making love to you; this simple technique gives you a lot more 'bulk' inside a loose vagina.

Q My vaginal muscles have been slack since the children were born, and this is affecting our love-making.

I know you have mentioned exercises to get these muscles back to normal. Can you recommend any literature which explains these? Also, is there a self-help group for women with this problem, which I believe is common?

A It sure is, ma'am! In fact, my postbag is full of letters on this subject.

Many gyms and women's aerobics classes now offer a course of pelvic floor muscle re-education. The basic exercises are explained on page 94. By the way, I recently encountered a journalist who asked me if pelvic floor exercises were so called because you did them on the floor!

Q Some friends invited my husband and me to a nude party in their indoor swimming pool. Things got a bit out of hand, and I made love with several guys in the water. What I am worried about is, could the chlorine in the pool have damaged my vagina?

A I'm assuming this letter isn't a hoax – since I see it was posted in the Surrey stockbroker belt, where sex in the swimming pool seems to be as socially acceptable as smoked salmon and Sainsbury's Soave.

I'd have said that chlorine is the least of your problems – for I know of no evidence that it damages a woman's innards. But if you go on having orgies in the indoor pool, you are in some danger of (a) pregnancy of unknown origin; (b) drowning.

The Vas Deferens

The *vas deferens* is the tube which brings sperms up from the testicle towards the penis. A man normally has two of these tubes: a few blokes have three, but this *isn't* an advantage to them, as we'll see in a moment.

The *vas* looks very like a thin piece of spaghetti. It can be felt with the fingertips through the skin of a man's scrotum (gently, please!) as – it runs up towards the groin.

But the reason why there's such a lot of interest in the *vas* these days is that it's the bit they chop when they do vasectomies.

This fantastically popular operation just involves making two tiny incisions in the skin of the scrotum – and then working via them to cut through each *vas*, and then tie the ends off.

Why are men who have a third *vas* at a disadvantage? Because the surgeon probably won't realise they have an extra *vas deferens*, and will fail to cut it. So, in their cases, the vasectomy won't work!

Happily, the sperm test which is done a couple of months or so after a vasectomy will detect the fact that there's another *vas deferens*, still sending up vast supplies of spermatozoa. The third *vas* can then be cut and tied off too.

Cutting through the *vas deferens* doesn't interfere with a man's production of sex hormones, or with his virility. It just gives him a great feeling of confidence that he's no longer exposing his female partner to the risk of unwanted pregnancy.

And that, of course, can make a *vas deferens* to his love life . . .

137

Vasectomy

While I was preparing this book, I was a bit disturbed to read that vasectomy had just been declared a crime in Italy. Yes – it's now a criminal offence, for both surgeon *and* patient! Presumably tourists with vasectomies will still be allowed in: at least, I hope so – because I happen to have had one.

In most civilised countries, however (especially those where the *machismo* tradition is dying), vasectomy has become fantastically popular in recent years. Surgeons find it hard to keep up with the demand, and it has almost become a matter of routine for the younger middle-aged man to consider getting himself vasectomised, to spare his wife the health risks of more years on the Pill or the IUD.

Among medical families in Britain, a recent study showed that about a quarter now rely on either vasectomy or female sterilisation as their method of contraception (with a 50/50 split between the two methods).

A vasectomy is really a very simple business indeed – and far less complex and traumatic than female sterilisation because the 'plumbing' is all external. The operation is often done under local anaesthetic – and indeed, I watched my own being done (though I wouldn't recommend this to the faint hearted).

In the few days after the operation the man can expect a fair amount of bruising and swelling. He should wear a support, and may need to take some pain-killers. He should definitely *not* undertake any heavy work (lifting, etc.) for several days.

There are a few complications, such as the occasional stitch slipping, leading to bleeding or a large but temporary swelling. Inevitably, this happened to *me* – and I had to spend about three weeks in bed. For full horrendous details, see Dr Richard Gordon's best-seller *Great Medical Disasters* (London: Heinemann Books).

But I've never known anybody come to any long-term harm

Q My sister's baby died after her husband had a vasectomy. What are his chances of reversing it?

A I'm so sorry to hear about this. Your brother-in-law's best bet would be to see the consultant urologist at a Medical School.

from a vasectomy. Unusually for surgical operations, no deaths have *ever* been reported —except for two tragic cases of lockjaw, which occurred in two men who were operated on in insanitary conditions in India.

Happily, a couple can resume love-making as soon as they like after the operation (some have been known to manage it about 2½ hours afterwards!). The man will not be 'safe', however, until he has had – on average – about a dozen climaxes, to clear out all the sperm in the upper part of his piping.

Surgeons recommend a simple sperm test, usually carried out two or three months after the operation, to make sure that no sperm is left in the fluid. Until then, the couple should use another method of contraception.

Yes, there *is* fluid produced – effectively the same volume as before. And yes – sex is just as good afterwards as it was previously.

However, men with psycho-sexual problems should be screened out by the counselling sessions provided before a vasectomy – partly because a man who has deep fears of castration may mistakenly get the idea that the operation has lessened his potency, or affected him in other ways.

Finally, if as a couple you decide on this method, there is one other thing you should bear in mind. It is this: *do not go in for it if you think you might change your mind.*

In general, it is best to regard vasectomy as an irreversible step. There *is* an operation to reverse it, but the results are not very good. So both of you should be very sure that vasectomy is the right *permanent solution to the question of contraception in your relationship.*

Note: No operation has a 100% success rate, and there are very rare cases in which a man fathers a child long after an apparently successful vasectomy.

He may be willing to attempt a reversal. But the 'pregnancy rate' is often well below 50%.

Because the results of vasectomy reversal are so unimpressive, cou-ples who are contemplating having hubby sterilised should bear in mind that it is possible to take out 'insurance' by depositing sperm in a private sperm bank.

VASECTOMY

Q My husband had a vasectomy some years ago, and we have made love without any protection since then. But he says that he has recently read reports of vasectomies failing after many years – and women getting pregnant as a result. Is this true?

A Well, nothing (including vasectomy) is ever 100% effective. It's true that there have been recent headlines about surgeons getting into trouble for failing to warn men about this ('Top Docs Face Sex Rap').

Every male who has a vasectomy should have one or (preferably) two sperm tests a few months after the operation, to make sure that he's not fertile. If this is done, then the couple can assume that the chance of further sperms finding their way through the bloke's blocked-up plumbing is fairly remote.

In practice, there's a general feeling that many (if not most) pregnancies which occur after a vasectomy are due to the well-known 'Milkman Syndrome'.

Q My husband is having trouble in getting a vasectomy because our doctor is violently opposed to anyone having the operation. Could we get it done privately?

A Certainly. There are now many private surgeons and clinics who do this astonishingly popular op. For instance, your husband could talk to the Marie Stopes Clinic in London (01-388 2585), which has always specialised in low-cost vasectomies. (I had my own done there.) It's a snip at about £100!

Q My husband had a vasectomy about 12 years ago, toward the end of his first marriage. After his divorce, he met me and we got married and have enjoyed a good relationship ever since. Would there be any chance of reversing the vasectomy, so that we could have children of our own?

A The chances of successful vasectomy reversal are not great, I'm afraid. But some intrepid surgeons – particularly in teaching hospitals – are willing to have a bash at this difficult and challenging operation.

The type of surgeon you and your husband need to consult is a urologist. They're a bit thin on the ground, but as it happens there is one at the large hospital in the town from which you write.

Venereal Diseases

VD is common nowadays, particularly among young adults. Anyone who has had a casual sexual liaison would be well advised to go to a hospital 'Genito-Urinary Clinic' for a check-up, *under conditions of strict confidentiality*. A few simple tests carried out there will tell whether infection has taken place. (These clinics are advertised quite widely nowadays. If you're in doubt, ring the nearest large hospital and enquire when the next 'Special Clinic' will be held, or call the Family Planning Information Service at 01-636 7866.)

It's important to bear in mind that VD in women (and occasionally men) may well produce no obvious symptoms. Therefore, if you have the least suspicion of it, have a check at once. Treatment, if carried out right away, is usually curative.

Prevention

VD is virtually always passed on by having sexual contact (though not necessarily actual intercourse) with an infected person. Repeated contact is not necessary — a few seconds can give it to you.

It's obvious, therefore, that VD would be rapidly wiped out in a world in which everybody was always faithful to his or her sexual partner. Blatant promiscuity, or 'sleeping around', is very likely to lead to infection, particularly in cities, large towns, and ports, where the incidence of VD is always high. Unfortunately, 'new' infections like herpes and AIDS are beginning to spread alarmingly in such areas.

In Britain, and some other countries, it's been shown statistically that a man who goes with street prostitutes is virtually certain to get VD before long.

Wearing a sheath and washing carefully immediately after intercourse provides at least some protection against venereal infection, but not much; it's far more sensible to avoid 'sleeping around'.

If you suspect that infection has occurred, cease all sexual activity at once in case you spread the disease further. If the clinic finds that you actually *do* have VD, you'll probably be given tracing slips to give to anyone you've slept with recently. Though it's embarrassing, always pass these on: otherwise the consequences for these people (and their future sexual contacts) may be disastrous.

Q I live in the Arabian Gulf, and a friend of mine is desperate to have her virginity restored by the operation you recently mentioned in SHE. My friend gave her virginity to the boy she loved at age 16. But now she must be a virgin in order to be married.

We are visiting England soon, and she could have the operation then. But you have said that there are some incompetent plastic surgeons in Britain. So who should she contact? Please help — you're our last hope.

A Your 'friend' wouldn't happen to be yourself love, would it?

Anyway, I think that the best thing to do would be to write to the British Association of Aesthetic Plastic Surgeons, c/o The Royal College of Surgeons, *35, Lincoln's Inn Fields, London WC2*. The operation is expensive. But I hope it will achieve the desired effect on the wedding night.

Q I read what you wrote in SHE about how women shouldn't feel that their vulvas were ugly or abnormal. Well, I'm not happy about the appearance of

mine, because the labia are far too long.

I would like to get them operated on before the summer holidays. Is this possible?

A What sort of summer holidays are you going on, I ask myself! Well ma'am, you'd have to get your skates on in order to have your labia shortened by bikini-time, but it can be done.

Though I honestly wouldn't recommend this op for most people, I am told by a cosmetic surgeon that there is a procedure which is known in the plastic surgery trade as a 'fanny-plasty'. It costs around a thousand quid, and it's possible to get it done through the British Association of Aesthetic Plastic Cosmetic Surgeons, mentioned left.

Please note that I *cannot* guarantee the results of such an operation to re-shape your vulva, though I quite understand your reasons for asking about it. After all, as Keats says in *Endymion,* 'A thing of beauty is a joy for ever. . .'

Q I feel that my sex organs are terribly ugly because my labia minora project through the labia majora.

I am too embarrassed to go to the doctor about this, but could I possibly have an operation to put it right?

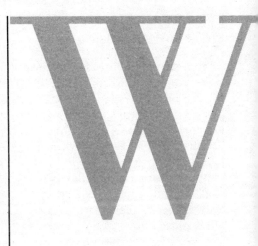

A The recent Delvin Report survey showed that quite a high proportion of women are unhappy about the appearance of their vulvas.

From your very clear and concise description I think you may actually be *normal*, but if you're badly distressed about the way you look, then certainly an operation is possible.

The vulva 'tidying-up' op usually costs somewhere in the region of a £1,000 surgeon's fee, plus hospital charges for your stay.

I really do think you should go to your doc's straight away and let him/her have a look at you to see if the operation is a reasonable idea to give you peace of mind.

Q I'm 43 and have recently developed a curious lump on the side of my vulva. My husband wants me to go to the doctor, but surely this isn't necessary?

A I beg you to have this checked out *immediately*. Unexplained lumps or ulcers on the vulva – particularly in the over-40s – demand an urgent medical opinion.

The Womb

The average woman's womb is only about as big as her clenched fist. It's very like a small pear, turned upside down, with the tip of the pear representing the cervix, or neck of the womb. The womb is actually a little bag of muscle which is powerful enough to push a baby out – and it's the contraction of this muscle fibre which produces the pains of labour. However, the womb is not all muscle. There's a thin lining, which is shed every month when a woman has her period.

Disorders

There are very many disorders of the womb. This is one reason for the fact that about one out of every five women eventually has her womb removed.

The main disorders are:

Fibroids. Benign swellings which develop in the muscular wall. Incredibly common, particularly in the over-thirties and in women who haven't had children. The cause is unknown and the symptoms are pain, or heavy periods, or difficulty in passing urine. If they don't cause symptoms, they can usually be left alone. Troublesome fibroids may have to be 'shelled out' or a hysterectomy may be necessary.

Prolapse. Prolapse of the womb means that it comes down into the vagina, and may even come outside. It's caused by weakening of the supports of the womb during childbirth. It is curable by a repair operation, or if necessary a hysterectomy.

Endometriosis. Painful nodules in the wall of the womb, and elsewhere in the pelvis. Treatable with hormones or, if necessary, surgical removal.

Cancer of the womb lining. Womb cancer (which is quite different from cancer of the cervix) kills about 1,000 British women each year. It usually starts in the womb lining, and can be triggered off by excessive stimulation with oestrogens. This is most common in women who have passed the menopause – and the giveaway symptom is *bleeding occurring after the menopause.* This must *always* be investigated. Cure is possible by hysterectomy.

Unfortunately, there is as yet no widely available screening test for cancer of the womb. Smear tests (for cancer of the cervix) do *not* detect cancer of the womb. There is a test, called 'out-patient curettage', but at the moment cost prevents it from being widely used.